The Pract
Manager
Visual Impairment

Design & Layout: Jane Hancock
Yellow Duck Creative
www.yellowduckcreative.com

Indexing: Christine Boylan PhD MCOptom

The Practical Management of Visual Impairment

Jane Macnaughton FCOptom Prof Cert LV

Dept of Ophthalmology, Leicester Royal Infirmary, Leicester, UK.
Nuffield Health Leicester Hospital, UK

Foreword by:
Professor Martin Rubinstein PhD FCOptom
Dept of Ophthalmology, Leicester Royal Infirmary, Leicester, UK.
Honorary Professor, School of Life and Health Sciences, Aston University, Birmingham, UK.

Clinical Editor:
Dr. Sandip Doshi PhD MCOptom
Optometrist East Sussex, UK

CLEARVIEW TRAINING

www.clearviewtraining.co.uk | 2018

Published by CLEARVIEW Training

First published 2018
ISBN 978 1 9998228 0 4

British Library Cataloguing in Publication Data

A catalogue record for this book is available from the British Library

Library of Congress Cataloging in Publication Data

A catalog record for this book is available from the Library of Congress

Note:
No reader should act on the basis of material contained within this publication without first taking professional advice appropriate to their particular circumstances. Neither the authors, editors or publisher assume any responsibility for any loss, injury or damage to persons or property arising from the materials contained within this book. Neither the authors, editors or publisher assume any responsibility for any errors or omissions within this book. It is the responsibility of the eyecare or treating practitioner to determine the best treatment or management of the patient. As new research impacts upon the methods of low vision services and practice, it is assumed that equipment, strategies and devices will change. The reader or practitioner is therefore advised to check the most current information.

VIPs, patients, clients or service users?

As times change so do the phrases we use within healthcare. Some terms that were once in common use, such as 'handicapped' for example have mostly disappeared. The majority of healthcare professionals currently use the term 'patient'. Rehabilitation workers and those working in the provision of social care may use the term 'clients,' 'service users' or 'members'. There are several terms used in the work of low vision. For convenience, the term 'patient' will be used throughout this text with no intended partiality or discrimination. In time this term may also change. Readers must be guided by what is considered the current correct phraseology.

Contents

Acknowledgements

As an optometrist and as a low-vision practitioner, my personal knowledge and experience have benefitted greatly from working alongside other professionals as part of a growing multidisciplinary profession. Rehabilitation workers, associated healthcare professionals, academics, service providers and volunteers, many of whom are themselves visually impaired, have enriched my experience in working in such a rewarding area of clinical practice. I have captured many of their individual comments, tips and experiences and have included them throughout this book.

My particular thanks go to **Stuart Baldwin** of Associated Optical, who has provided most of the images or equipment for the illustrations throughout this text. Stuart has given me endless opportunities in recent years to teach and to impart my enthusiasm for low vision practice to fellow practitioners on the value of good quality, well-designed products.

I am indebted to **Keziah Latham**, who has contributed to this text by writing the chapter on The Impact of Visual Impairment and Rehabilitation. Kez is a key driver in UK low vision research and her influence spreads across several chapters. I am further indebted to **Rasmeet Chadha**, who was persuaded into writing the chapter on the Assessment of Children and Young People with Low Vision whilst on maternity leave. An experienced hospital optometrist, I share Rasmeet's enthusiasm for working with the younger age groups and have turned to her many times for opinion and advice.

Thank you to **Jane Hancock** of yellowduckcreative.co.uk who has designed and set the entire layout of the book and who showed incredible patience throughout a multitude of corrections.

And finally, my gratitude extends to clinical editor and longstanding friend, **Sandip Doshi**. Sandip and I embarked upon our journey into optometry together of which at the time of writing, has now slipped into its fourth decade.

My gratitude also extends to the following colleagues and friends who have cast their eyes over the content of this book. All are experienced and dedicated low vision practitioners and who share my passion for working in this field:

David Adams BSc PhD MCOptom
Mary Bairstow BSc MCOptom
Andy Cook FBDO (Hons) LVA
Helen Denton FBDO (Hons) LVA Prof Cert LV
Sandip Doshi BSc PhD MCOptom
David Elks BSc MCOptom
Ronak Gosai BSc (Hons) DipHE
Louise Gow BSc MSc OD MCOptom
Cilla Hubbard FBDO Prof Cert LV
Zahra Jessa BSc PhD MCOptom
Keziah Latham BSc PhD FCOptom Prof Cert LV FHEA
Kevin McNally FBDO (Hons) LVA BSc MCOptom
Annette Parkinson BSc PhD MCOptom Prof Cert LV FHEA
Martin Rubinstein BSc PhD FCOptom
Barbara Ryan BSc PhD MCOptom Prof Cert Glauc
Rebecca Scott Rehabilitation Services Co-ordinator
Adrian Sexton BSc MCOptom Prof Cert Glauc Prof Cert LV Higher Cert LV
Nilpa Shah BSc PhD MCOptom

For help with additional photographs, equipment and diagrams:

Alev, Cherry, Emma, Sibbo, Fiona and Jennifer, from Vista, Leicester, UK
Stuart Baldwin, Associated Optical, UK
Paul, David and Alex Brook, Scalford, UK
Mark Bullimore, Ridgevue Publishing, USA
Neil Guest, Anglia Ruskin University, UK
Bill Harvey, Optometrist, UK
Ian Hughes and Nick Hamlett, Associated Optical, UK
Fiona McCormick, Fife Society for the Blind, UK
Louise Pearson, Barclays UK
Hannah Scoones, Band-it, UK
Nilpa Shah, Moorfields Eye Hospital, London, UK

A note about magnification

The understanding of the concepts of magnification is important if we are to give our patients the best advice on the aids and devices that produce enlargement. However, magnification is one of the most misunderstood terms in low vision practice and is often over-complicated by those of us who work in the industry, making it difficult for students and practitioners new to the subject area to understand.

Nigel Slater renowned cook, presenter and author,*

> *"There is too much talk of cooking being an art or a science – we are only making ourselves something to eat "*

Whilst the mathematical concepts of magnification are undoubtedly essential, it must be remembered that all we are trying to do is improve the visibility of an object by making it bigger. In simplest terms, magnification is relative; a simple comparison of the new image size to the old one before magnification was introduced – a before and after effect.

Therefore, magnification must be taken in the context to which it is intended. The most important message throughout this text is that real patients using magnification for real-world activities will all perform differently. Variations in the effect of magnification are caused by how the device is used, from the power of the patient's habitual prescription, to how far the magnifier is held away from both the eye and the page.

Thus, calculating how much magnification or enlargement a patient needs is merely a starting point with which to base your assessment and what practitioners need to understand is how to make the most appropriate adjustments for each situation as they arise so that the patient can get the most out of the aid. Ultimately all magnification devices are a compromise and one that some patients will manage wholly, in part or perhaps not at all.

*Real Cooking, Nigel Slater, 1997 Penguin Books

Dedication

This book I dedicate to my patients at Vista, Leicestershire and Rutland's leading charity for people with sight loss, many of whom have had their lives turned upside down by vision loss. They have welcomed me into their homes to disclose the practical and emotional challenges they face on a daily basis so that they could give something back to help improve the quality of our low vision services for the benefit of others.

Jane Macnaughton

Foreword

Visual impairment is the consequence of a disease or abnormality affecting the function of the visual system. This is predominantly the result of genetic factors or an acquired disease process notably due to ageing, as a manifestation of systemic disease or trauma. Such impairment results in limitations in the activities that an individual can undertake or complete and thus may restrict that individual's participation in society. The level of impairment can be assessed by a variety of methods which measure visual function.

In modern clinical and social care, the concept of 'quality of life' (especially 'health-related' and 'vision-related' assessment measures) is a recognised index of the impact of visual impairment. This is often used to guide professionals in optimising care and advice for the individual.

As a result of the increasing longevity of the population, particularly in the developed world, the impact of age-related causes of visual impairment is becoming ever more significant. Despite phenomenal advances in medical and surgical treatments in clinical ophthalmology, optical and optometric approaches to the management of visual impairment remain the mainstay of care. This care is best provided by a multi-disciplinary team combining clinical, social and rehabilitation support individualised to the particular person.

This book provides a very comprehensive and, importantly for the busy professional, a very practical approach to the entire subject. The twelve chapters cover topics including definitions and epidemiology, the impact of visual impairment, clinical assessment of both adults and children, magnification and optical and non-optical devices.

The layout of the book is impressively clear and straightforward. The use of bullet point lists and highlighted boxes giving clinical examples draws the reader's attention to important information and facilitates identification of the key issues and facts.

Whether the reader is a clinician or not there are many practical suggestions here for everyone. As befits the title, the emphasis is very much patient-focussed, and there is a modern and contemporary approach to the subject matter. As such this book provides a very useful resource for all eyecare and other professionals involved in the management of visual impairment.

Trainees and students will also find this book both easy to read and a very informative resource.

Jane Macnaughton is a highly respected optometrist who has many years' experience as a low vision practitioner. She works in clinical practice in both hospital and private settings and is an active contributor to academic and educational arenas.

Contributors: Rasmeet Chadha is a recognised authority on paediatric visual impairment and Keziah Latham has a strong track record in both clinical and academic low vision practice.

Martin P Rubinstein

"I've always loved change, and this is certainly a change. It's quite exciting, really. I'm trying to work out how to turn it to my advantage. I will, you know."

Sue Townsend, speaking to The Guardian in 2001

CHAPTER ONE

Definitions & Epidemiology of Visual Impairment

“Despite major clinical and technological advancements, there are many people, both young and old, who will not have their sight fully restored. Comprehensive low vision services recognise that the majority of these people have some vision that can be enhanced and successfully utilised for tasks that require vision.”

Mary Bairstow, BSc MCOptom, Vision UK

Definitions & Epidemiology of Visual Impairment

ICF: The International Classification of Functioning, Disability and Health

The World Health Organisation (WHO) first published a trial document in 1980 called the International Classification of Impairment, Disability and Handicap.[1] The purpose of the document was to provide a framework for the description of health and health-related states. In 2001, the document became known as the International Classification of Functioning, Disability and Health, or ICF, and was officially endorsed by all WHO Member states as the international standard to describe and measure health and disability. The document provides tools to understand the health of a population and how individuals interact with their environment. The ICF also provides a framework for healthcare services that may be used to measure health outcomes and monitor the effectiveness of interventions.[2] (See also chapter 12).

Global estimates of visual impairment

90% of those suffering from a visual impairment live in developing countries. The WHO estimates that there are over 280 million people suffering from a visual impairment, with approximately 246 million classified as having 'low vision,' as defined in Table 1.1, and 39 million classified as 'blind.' With 90% of the world's visually impaired currently living in low-income settings, low vision is a significant socioeconomic burden. Furthermore, the WHO estimates that 80% of all visual impairment is either preventable or may be cured.[3–6]

Definitions of blindness, low vision and visual impairment

Table 1.1 shows the World Health Organisation's ICD-10 categories of severity of visual impairment recommended by the Resolution of the International Council of Ophthalmology and the Recommendations of the WHO Consultation on "Development of standards for characterisation of vision loss and visual functioning.[7,8] Moderate visual impairment combined with severe visual impairment is grouped under the term low vision and low vision taken together with blindness represents all visual impairment.

The definitions of visual impairment vary across the world, which makes comparisons between populations difficult. Previously, estimates of blindness and low vision were based upon "best-corrected" vision, however, there is evidence that uncorrected refractive error is a significant global burden and thus updates on population-based studies of visual impairment cannot overlook this significant contribution to the epidemiology of visual impairment. Consequently, definitions of WHO visual impairment are now based upon "presenting"(i.e. habitual) vision/visual acuity. [8]

The causes of global visual impairment and blindness (as defined by the WHO)

Globally, the principal causes of **visual impairment** are uncorrected refractive errors (43%) and cataract (33%). Other causes are glaucoma (2%), age-related macular degeneration, diabetic retinopathy, trachoma and corneal opacities, all approximately 1%. A large proportion of causes (18%) are undetermined.[4,5,9]

The causes of **blindness** are cataract (51%), glaucoma (8%), age-related macular degeneration (5%), childhood blindness and corneal opacities (4%), uncorrected refractive errors and trachoma (3%), and diabetic retinopathy (1%). The undetermined causes are 21%.[4]

Table 1.1 ICD-10 categories of severity of visual impairment[8]
(**Note:** LogMAR conversions are given for reference although these do not appear in the original document).

Presenting distance visual acuity*			
Category		**Worse than:**	**Equal to or better than:**
Normal Vision	0 Mild or no visual impairment		6/18 20/70 LogMAR 0.48
Low Vision	1 Moderate visual impairment	6/18 20/70 LogMAR 0.48	6/60 20/200 LogMAR 1.0
	2 Severe visual impairment	6/60 20/200 LogMAR 1.0	3/60 20/400 LogMAR 1.3
Blind	3 Blindness **	3/60 20/400 LogMAR 1.3	1/60 20/1200 LogMAR 1.8
	4 Blindness ***	1/60 20/1200 LogMAR 1.8	Light perception
	5 Blindness	No perception of light	
	9	Undetermined or unspecified	

* Where visual acuity is measured with presenting correction, if any.
** If the extent of the visual field is taken into account, patients with a visual field in the better eye of no greater than 10^{0} but greater than 5^{0} in radius around central fixation should be placed under category 3.
***Patients with a visual field of no greater than 5^{0} are placed in category 4 (even when central visual acuity is not impaired).

Age and visual impairment

Approximately 20% of the world's population is over the age of 50. With an ageing population, the rise of visual impairment as a consequence of age-related conditions is evident in developed countries. Globally the WHO estimates that 65% of all people who have a visual impairment are over the age of 50.[3]

Age-related macular degeneration (AMD) affects approximately 9% of the global population and is most prevalent among individuals with European ancestry.[10] In the United Kingdom, AMD is the leading cause of visual impairment, with glaucoma, hereditary retinal disorders, cerebrovascular disease and diabetes adding significant contributions.[11] In the United States, approximately 0.4% of the general population has late or advanced AMD with the prevalence of advanced AMD rising to 8% among those 75 years of age and older.[12] Global projections suggest that 196 million individuals worldwide will be suffering from AMD by 2020 due to the rapid and consistent growth of the ageing population.[10] Recent projections estimate that worldwide the number of individuals with AMD will reach 196 million in 2020 and 288 million in 2040.[10]

VISION 2020 was launched in 1999 by the World Health Organisation together with more than 20 international non-governmental organisations involved in eyecare and prevention and management of blindness that comprise the International Agency for the Prevention of Blindness (IAPB). The VISION 2020 mission has been to eliminate the main causes of all preventable and treatable blindness as a public health issue by the year 2020.

There were three major objectives:

- To raise the profile of the causes of avoidable blindness and the solutions that will help to eliminate the problem.
- To identify and secure the necessary resources around the world in order to provide an increased level of prevention and treatment programmes.
- To facilitate the planning, development and implementation of the three core VISION 2020 strategies by National Programmes.

Core strategies to deliver these objectives have been:

- **Disease control:** facilitate the implementation of specific programmes to control and treat the major causes of blindness.

- **Human resource development:** support training of ophthalmologists and other eyecare personnel to provide eyecare.
- **Infrastructure and appropriate technology development:** assist to improve infrastructure and technology to make eyecare more available and accessible.

Visual impairment in children

The WHO estimates 19 million children worldwide are living with a visual impairment, 60% of which is due to uncorrected refractive error.[3] The correction of refractive error has been one of the priorities of the Global Initiative for the Elimination of Avoidable Blindness known as VISION 2020, the Right to Sight.[13–15]

The major causes of blindness and visual impairment in children are largely determined by socioeconomic regional differences. The level of support that families and children have will also impact upon their long-term development. In middle and high-income countries, conditions of the central nervous system and optic nerve together with retinopathy of prematurity are major causes of visual impairment, whereas in countries with low socioeconomic status, the corneal complications subsequent to measles, or Vitamin A deficiency are significant causes. In half of the children who are severely visually impaired the cause could certainly have been preventable and treatable.[16,17]

Associated comorbidities

Visual impairment in older patients has been found to have a broad range of both physical and mental health comorbidities compared to those of the same age without visual impairment, with high rates of multiple comorbidities. This has implications for both low vision and rehabilitation services to meet the more complex needs of patients with additional disability.[18–20]

Anxiety & Depression

Large-scale epidemiologic studies indicate that over 30% of people with a visual impairment have significant depressive symptoms, which is 3 times higher than in the general population.[20,21] How individuals cope with long-term adjustment to sight loss will vary due to a wide variety of underlying factors such as personality type, disease process and level of psychological and rehabilitative support, with some able to adjust better than others. However, a large number find the practical problems associated with sight loss overwhelming.

Whilst both the screening and treatment of depression and anxiety is often beyond the professional scope of practice of many low vision practitioners, it is important to remain sensitive and be able to ask probing questions to determine whether onward referral for suitable support and management is required. Chapter 12 outlines this in more detail.

Summary

Although many different definitions of visual impairment are used for the purpose of legislation throughout the world, one of the main purposes of defining and categorising visual impairment is to identify those in need of support; to structure and deliver appropriate services according to need and to provide a framework for future services.

The WHO continues to work to eliminate avoidable blindness and increase rehabilitation for people with residual visual impairment or who are blind. Building accessible and inclusive health systems have been a major focus since the turn of the century.

References

1. World Health Organisation. International Classification of impairments, disabilites and handicaps (ICIDH). 1980;(May 1976).
2. World Health Organisation, World Health Organisation G. The International classification of functioning, disability and health. 2013;18:237.
3. World Health Organisation. Visual impairment and blindness. Factsheet No 282. World Health Organisation; 2014.
4. Pascolini D, Mariotti SP. Global estimates of visual impairment: 2010. Br J Ophthalmol. 2012 May;96(5):614–8.
5. Stevens GA, White RA, Flaxman SR, Price H, Jonas JB, Keeffe J, et al. Global prevalence of vision impairment and blindness: Magnitude and temporal trends, 1990-2010. Ophthalmology. 2013;120(12):2377–84.
6. Bourne RR, Stevens G, White RA, Flaxman S, Mascarenhas M, Price H, et al. The Global Burden of Disease Study: the Impact of Vision Loss: prevalence and trends of blindness and visual impairment over the past 28 years. Invest Ophthalmol Vis Sci. 2012;53(14):3175–3175.
7. World Health Organisation. ICD-10 International statistical classification of diseases and related health problems, 1994.
8. World Health Organisation. ICD-10 Update 2006.
9. Naidoo KS, Leasher J, Bourne RR, Flaxman SR, Jonas JB, Keeffe J, et al. Global vision impairment and blindness due to uncorrected refractive error, 1990-2010. Optom Vis Sci. 2016;93(3):227–34.
10. Wong WL, Su X, Li X, Cheung CMG, Klein R, Cheng CY, et al. Global prevalence of age-related macular degeneration and disease burden projection for 2020 and 2040: A systematic review and meta-analysis. Lancet Glob Heal. 2014;2(2).
11. Quartilho A, Simkiss P, Zekite A, Xing W, Wormald R, Bunce C. Leading causes of certifiable visual loss in England and Wales during the year ending 31 March 2013. Eye. 2016;44 (April 2015):1–6.
12. Friedman DS, O'Colmain BJ, Muñoz B, Tomany SC, McCarty C, DeJong PTVM, et al. Prevalence of age-related macular degeneration in the United States. Arch Ophthalmol. 2004; 122:564-572.
13. Dandona R, Dandona L. Socioeconomic status and blindness. Br J Ophthalmol. 2001;85(12):1484–8.

14. Vision 2020: The Right to Sight: A global initiative to eliminate avoidable blindness. Arch Ophthalmol. 2004;122(4):615–20.

15. World Health Organisation. Blindness: Vision 2020 - The global initiative for the elimination of avoidable blindness. WHO fact sheet. 2015.

16. Gilbert C, Foster A. Childhood blindness in the context of VISION 2020 - The right to sight. Bulletin World Health Organ. 2001;79(3):227–32.

17. Kong L, Fry M, Al-Samarraie M, Gilbert C, Steinkuller PG. An update on progress and the changing epidemiology of causes of childhood blindness worldwide. J AAPOS. 2012;16(6):501–7.

18. Court H, McLean G, Guthrie B, Mercer SW, Smith DJ. Visual impairment is associated with physical and mental comorbidities in older adults: a cross-sectional study. BMC Med. 2014 Jan 17;12(1):181.

19. Margrain TH, Nollett C, Shearn J, Stanford M, Edwards RT, Ryan B, et al. The depression in visual impairment trial (DEPVIT): trial design and protocol. BMC Psychiatry. 2012;12(1):57.

20. Nollett CL, Bray N, Bunce C V., Casten RJ, Edwards RT, Hegel MT, et al. High prevalence of untreated depression in patients accessing low vision services. Ophthalmology. 2016;123(2):440–1.

21. Evans J, Fletcher A, Wormald R. Depression and anxiety in visually impaired older people. Ophthalmology. 2007;114(2):283–8.

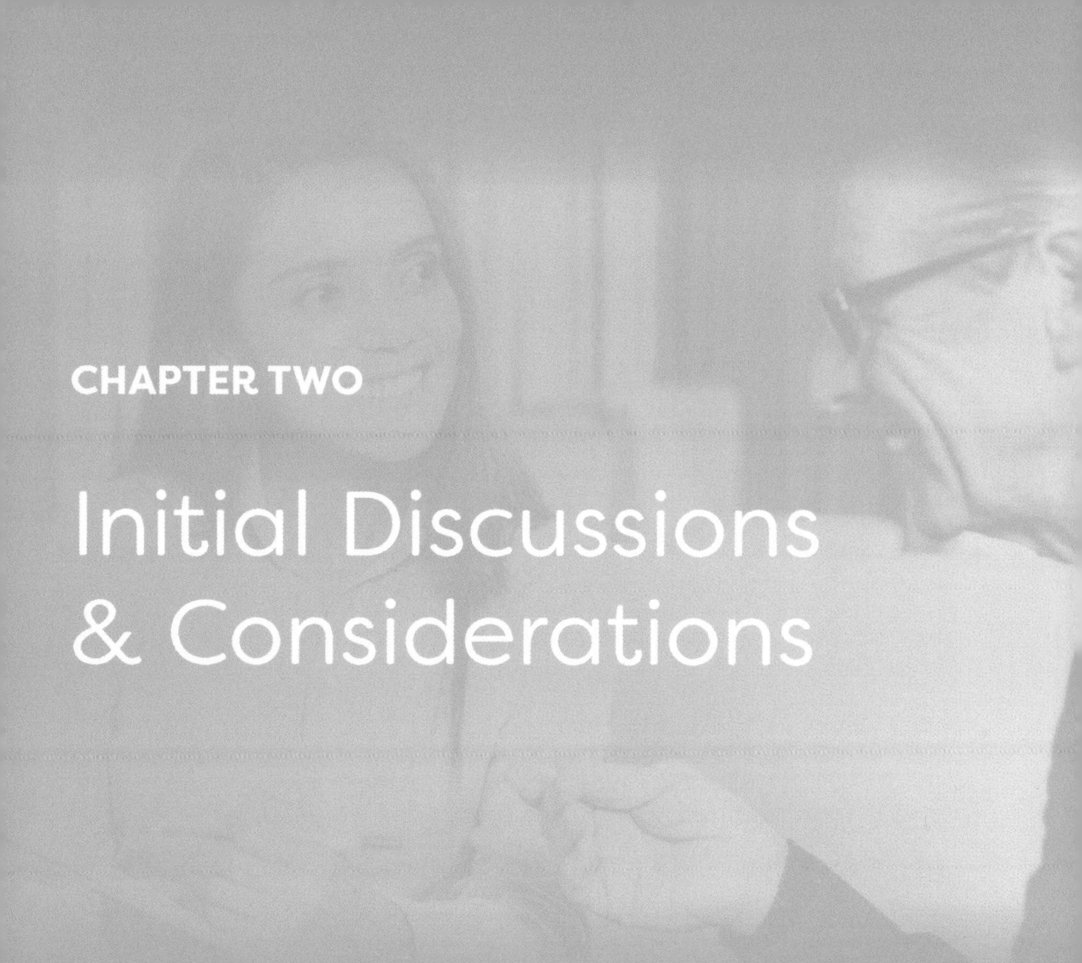

CHAPTER TWO

Initial Discussions & Considerations

"Many low vision patients have not been given a forum in which to explain their difficulties to a provider. The initial assessment is vital to establish trust between the patient and the practitioner in order for the patient to provide key information about their individual situation. This in turn will impact the quality of care provided."

Cilla Hubbard FBDO Prof Cert LV

Initial Discussions & Considerations

Introduction

The importance of a methodical and thorough discussion during the initial consultation cannot be underestimated. Patients have often seen many eyecare professionals before the low vision examination and may have had a complex history prior to vision loss. Whether the patient is still undergoing treatment or whether they have been discharged by their consultant, they may have come to the low vision assessment with a variety of preconceived ideas.

The practical implications that acquired vision loss has upon the performance of daily activities will vary between individuals. Furthermore, the disabling effect resulting from the inability to read, or the loss of independent mobility following the withdrawal of a driving licence, may lead to additional emotional consequences. Therefore, being able to assess the practical and psychosocial impact of vision loss at an individual level on entry to low vision services is fundamental before determining the most suitable device or rehabilitative service for each individual patient.[1–4]

During the opening discussion with the patient, it is important for practitioners to introduce themselves and explain the purpose of the low vision assessment. The patient may have seen several eyecare professionals by the time they reach the low vision clinic and may be apprehensive about the consultation. An initial introduction not only allows the practitioner to set the scene but help the patient to relax. It is also an opportunity to allow for a discussion on any unrealistic expectations the patient has about the purpose of the assessment.

The following section will deal with the initial discussion, the expectations of the patient and accompanying carers, the relevance of the detailed history taken and the importance of a detailed task analysis or assessment of needs. All such information gathering should be tailored to the patient's individual circumstance and so will vary from one person to the next. For example, in the case of children with a visual impairment, both school and home life will be discussed and similarly those who are working will need their working environment taken into consideration. Older patients who live alone may have different needs to those who live with a partner or family.

The impact of sight loss

A loss of visual function will have brought about significant lifestyle changes, such as the loss of a driver's licence. By establishing these from the outset, the practitioner can begin to address individual needs. Therefore, build a detailed picture of the patient's everyday life, and make a note to return to specific points when performing a more detailed task analysis. The lists below contain examples of the level of detail needed to conduct a low vision assessment; a structured initial discussion goes a long way in understanding the very personal nature the impact of sight loss has had on the patient's lifestyle and wellbeing. Use both open and closed questions and ensure that enough time is allowed so that detail may be discussed and recorded and to allow the patient to gain confidence in the process.

Level of vision and effect upon daily living

Patients often feel the need to describe in detail what they can and cannot see.

Example questions

- Describe your vision to me. For example, if I sit directly in front of you can you describe me in any detail at all?
- Do you find it easier to look to the side of things to be able to catch a glimpse of them better?
- What happens when you try look to the side of something instead of directly at it?
- Can you describe to me what sort of problems you have been having since your vision deteriorated?
- For how long has your visual impairment been affecting you on a daily basis?
- How rapidly did your vision deteriorate?

Home, family and social support

Example questions

- Do you live alone?
- Do you have extra help?
- What local support do you have? Friends? Family, neighbours?
- Are you managing to take care of yourself?
- Are you able to read and reply to your own mail? Your own finances?
- Do you need to cook for yourself? How are you managing with cooking instructions and packets?
- Are you having difficulty with the cooker dials or the washing machine?
- How do you occupy the day?
- How well are you able to see the television?
- Are you able to see the subtitles on the television?
- Do you have any hobbies that have been impacted?
- Do you belong to any social groups?
- How do you get there?
- Have you told your friends you have a visual impairment?

Less familiar environments

Although not necessarily within the remit of a low vision practitioner, questions should ideally address the patient's current level of mobility, in particular whether the sight loss has impacted upon their ability to move about confidently out of doors or within unfamiliar environments.

Example questions

- Are you mobile? How mobile are you?
- Are you able to get out on your own?
- Has your sight loss affected your ability to go out of the house?
- Have you had any falls in the past year?
- Are you using public transport?

- Are you able to go shopping alone for food?
- How do you get there?
- Are you able to see the prices in the supermarket?
- Are you able to guide yourself about the aisles?
- Do you have trouble from glare out of doors? Indoors?

Work or education

Don't forget to ask all patients of any age if they are working, enrolled in educational courses or have a voluntary role. Questions relating to children and young people are covered in Chapter 11.

Example questions

- Are you working? What is the nature of your role?
- Has your vision loss impacted your role?
- How are you managing to get to work?
- Have you informed your employer/s?
- Have they been able to make changes to your role?
- Have you had any formal assessment at work for additional assistance or equipment for example?

The use of PROMs: structured assessment of needs

In recent years the development and use of patient reported outcome measures (PROMs) has expanded to include the assessment of vision related activity limitations. Evidence suggests that PROMs may provide more personalised commissioning of support that could enhance clinical care and reduce costs.[5] The uptake of PROMs has been steady across healthcare services, but perhaps less so within the visual rehabilitation sector. However their use, where appropriate, allows for a more patient-centred approach to low vision and rehabilitative assessment; for identifying and planning needs and to monitor the effectiveness of service outcomes. By using a systematic approach, PROMs such at the Participation and Activity Inventory, have been shown to more comprehensively identify the needs of people with visual impairment by preventing personal goals from being overlooked.[6,7] Chapter 12 discusses the use of PROMs in the assessment of rehabilitation and low vision needs.

Clinical history

Determine the disease process, previous or pending treatments and whether the vision has stabilised. Many patients, despite having been through the hospital system, have a poor understanding of the underlying condition that is causing the drop in their acuity. This may impact upon their motivation; if a patient believes that a pending treatment will reverse rather than stop the progression of the disease process, they may not be willing to try using a device in the short term.

Example questions

- What do you understand about your condition?
- How long has this been affecting you?
- How quickly did your vision deteriorate?
- Has it changed recently?
- Can you tell me what treatment you have already had?
- Do you have any pending treatment?
- When is your next appointment?
- Have you been discharged?

Charles Bonnet Syndrome

Patients suffering from acquired vision loss should be asked about Charles Bonnet Syndrome (CBS).[8] CBS consists of simple (e.g. flashes, floaters, shapes) or complex (e.g. animals, faces, objects) visual hallucinations in the absence of psychological or neurological disease and is widely accepted as being a relatively common condition that is under-reported by patients, often due to the fear of being labelled with mental illness or dementia.[9]

Often these hallucinations can be very vivid and detailed and can occur at any time with up to a third of patients describing the experience as disturbing, with a significant impact upon quality of life.[10] Studies on prevalence rates are highly variable and suggest that CBS may be as high as 60%.[11,12] Hallucinations can persist for many years, with a reported 75% of patients reporting symptoms of CBS for five years duration.[11]

CBS is particularly prevalent in age-related macular disease but has also been reported in patients with extensive visual field loss but who retain good central acuity. Although there's a growing research base into the condition, the underlying mechanism causing the hallucinations still remains a matter of debate.

What is clear is that practitioners should be asking about symptoms of CBS actively. A number of leaflets are now produced by various organisations to assist in the education of patients, carers and the wider healthcare community. But despite Charles Bonnet first describing his grandfather's hallucinations circa 1760,[13] the wider healthcare profession has been slow to catch on.

Whilst research continues to understand CBS and to find methods of reducing the frequency and duration of hallucinations, patients who meanwhile report a negative effect upon quality of life, an increase in associated fear, or a reduction in activities, should be signposted for assistance in coping strategies or alternative treatments in being able to live with the condition.[11,12]

Establish comorbidities

Detail should be sought regarding a general medical condition when it has a bearing on the use of a low vision device. For example, a patient whose hands are severely arthritic may have difficulty in using a hand-held device. Patients who already have reduced mobility as a result of arthritis may report that their vision loss further compounds their difficulties in moving about out of doors or in unfamiliar environments.

Emotional health

Acquired and irreversible vision loss is a life-changing event and a major cause of disability in the older population[14,15] and those affected may be confronted with a number of unwelcome practical and physical challenges arising from that loss. There is strong evidence linking acquired vision loss in the older population to an increased risk of mental health problems including depression and anxiety. Chapter 12 outlines the importance of establishing the possibility of underlying symptoms of depression or anxiety in patients with vision loss.

Previous rehabilitative and social care interventions

Inter-professional integration greatly improves the support and assistance of the help on offer to people with a visual impairment. Where reports are not available, establish whether or not the patient has been in contact with any other rehabilitative or social care professional. If it has been some time since a rehabilitation worker has been to visit the patient, a significant change in vision or change in personal circumstances, such as loss of a partner may indicate a follow up visit.

Example questions

- Have you had any contact with health and social care services locally?
- Have you had a home visit or did you attend a local centre for assistance?
- What assistance or equipment did they provide? Are they still in use?
- What other aids or useful equipment do you have in place?
- How long ago did you have the equipment installed?
- Has your vision changed again since that visit?
- Do you feel that you need to speak other people in a similar situation?
- Are you in touch with any local support groups or a befriending service?

A detailed task analysis

During the initial discussion start making a list of tasks that the patient has mentioned he is struggling with, especially if these tasks may be aided with additional light and magnification. Once the list is made of individual tasks, it is then important to discuss the significance or importance of each and determine whether the patient is disabled by the loss of function. For example, the inability to see a train indicator board may not hold any significance to the patient if he has no plans of using public transport on a regular basis. However, some patients may have stopped using public transport because they are no longer confident in doing so, rather than the fact that they have no special need to. On the other hand, the inability to see a computer screen will have obvious employment significance if the patient's job depends upon it.

In establishing the print size, quality and working distance, it is useful to have a variety of print samples available for use, including newspapers, puzzles, cooking instructions and large print books (Figure 2.1). When the task is quite specific, such as music sheets, or a favourite knitting pattern, then it is worth asking the patient to bring a sample of the print with them. If working with children or students, ask them to bring samples of their work including a textbook or exam paper.

Commonly reported near tasks

- Newsprint, TV listings
- Large print books
- Cooking instructions and sell-by dates
- Shop prices
- Packets in the supermarket
- Using coins and banknotes
- Signing a cheque
- Using an ATM, entering PIN numbers
- Mail, bank statements, writing Christmas or birthday cards
- Following a knitting pattern
- Taking tablets, eye-drops
- Keeping a diary, calendar
- Setting the cooker, washing machine or microwave dials
- Restaurant menus
- Dialing the telephone
- Using computer, tablet, smartphone

Commonly reported distance tasks

Below is a list of commonly reported distance tasks that may indicate the need for a distance magnification device, glare management or referral for assistance on mobility.

Figure 2.1 Patients regularly report difficulties with cooking instructions, sell-by dates, poor contrast and coloured print. It is useful to have a wide selection available when discussing difficulties and demonstrating devices.

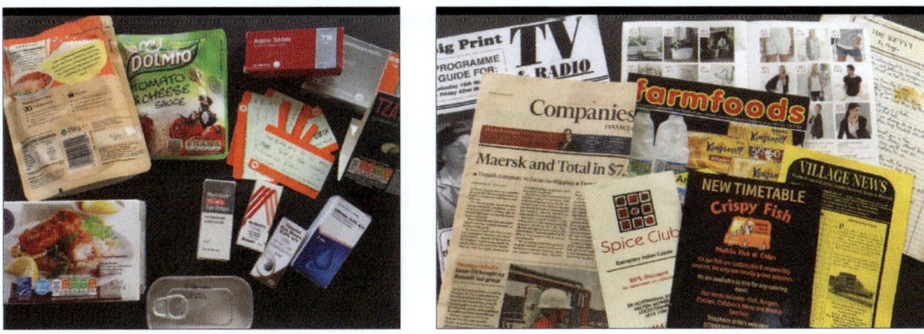

- Watching television
- Television subtitles, quiz show questions and answers
- Crossing a road
- Identifying buses, bus numbers
- Watching football, cricket, etc., at the grounds, or on the television
- Traveling on the trams or Underground
- Train indicator boards
- Shopping aisles in the supermarket
- Pavements, slopes and steps
- Stairs indoors, escalators

Task duration

Establish whether the task is either a

- 'Spot' or 'survival' reading task, such as setting the cooker dials or establishing a 'best before' date on food packaging.

- Fluent reading task, such a column of newspaper print

The length of time concentrating on a reading task will have a bearing on the strength of magnification prescribed and the type of device issued. For example, a patient who needs a device such as a hand magnifier to check the cooker dials will require different magnification and possibly a separate type of device for reading a large print book, even if the size of the task is the same. For fluent reading, a degree of acuity in reserve may be required as working near the acuity threshold will be too difficult or tiring for the patient and the outcome less likely to be successful[16–19] The importance of acuity and contrast reserves is discussed further in Chapter 5.

The previous lists are by no means exhaustive. The practitioner will be guided by the needs of the individual. A friend or family member may additionally assist the process if they are allowed to sit in on the consultation. However, it is important to set out expectations from the start. All low vision devices are a compromise to an individual who has previously had 'normal sight', and the use of these will be determined by several factors, such as the patient's level of motivation. Even the approach or the manner in which the practitioner manages the consultation will have an impact upon the outcome.

Therefore, at the end of the initial discussion the practitioner will have built up a picture of the patient's

Needs: size, working distance, location, position and duration of a series of tasks

Expectations: do they understand the compromise(s) that may be required to use a low vision device?

Motivation: a key to success

Additional considerations:

- Have they given up or will they try? Sadly, too many patients suffer in silence, often alone, under the misconception that there is nothing that can be done and that visual tasks are no longer achievable.
- If they say that they are not reading is it because they are not interested or is it because they cannot see well enough?
- Do not subscribe to stereotypes (many older patients are still working, wish to surf the internet, use tablets and have smartphones), so do not limit questions about expectations to assumed stereotypical age behaviour.

Current spectacles and low vision devices in current use

To be able to provide an improvement on the current device, it is worth establishing its limitations. Improvements may not be realistic, such as the regular request for providing a stronger magnifier, and one that covers the entire page. Ask the patient to bring the device to the consultation, even if it is no longer in use. Being able to compare it directly with others helps to restore confidence and keep expectations realistic.

Example questions

- Have you tried using a magnifier?
- Where/from whom did you get it?
- Do you find it useful?
- What can you manage to do with it?
- What can you not manage with it?
- Is there anything you can no longer do with it that you used to be able to?
- Has your vision worsened since you were prescribed or bought the device?
- Can you show me how you use it?
- Do you use it with or without your spectacles?
- If it were taken away, would you miss it?

It is therefore essential for the patient to bring all current spectacles and low vision aids to the assessment whether they are in use or not. If the patient has had a visual impairment for some time, then it is likely that they will have already tried using a magnifier. Even if it is one they used for stamp collecting 20 years ago, discuss its limitations: what can they or can they not do with it? It is a useful exercise to go through each device or pair of spectacles systematically; the practitioner may pick up additional information about managing expectations and the degree of patient motivation. Furthermore, it is not uncommon to find that a patient has been using an inappropriate spectacle correction with their current magnifier.

Record type, approximate age, condition and equivalent lens power of magnifier

- A full description is necessary for easy identification.
- Record specifically what each aid is used for
- Record its shortfall - ask the patient to feedback on how they use it and what difficulties they have with it
- Record level of vision achieved and the working distance where relevant.

Note: Magnification noted on the side of hand or stand devices may differ between manufacturers, occasionally termed as either 'trade' or 'nominal' magnification (Chapter 5). Therefore, many practitioners opt to record the equivalent lens power of the magnifier instead, which avoids confusion.

Signposting onto other services

Low vision practitioners rarely work in isolation. Many of the responses to the detailed questions above may not lie within the direct remit or responsibility of the low vision practitioner; however, at the end of the low vision assessment and at the point of concluding the consultation, practitioners should be able to discuss the need for further referral onto other associated professionals. For example, referral to the patient's general practitioner may be indicated if the patient is suffering from symptoms of depression; referral to a rehabilitation worker if the patient is struggling with activities of daily living within the home; for mobility, cane or trailing techniques or to a falls clinic if the patient is struggling with poor mobility. Early intervention is the key for successful outcomes from many services and the low vision practitioner is encouraged to have a good understanding of what other services are available. The practical management of low vision therefore is not a stand-alone service but part of a wider rehabilitation process to improve the patient's independence and quality of life.

References

1. Heyl V, Wahl H. Psychosocial adaptation to age-related vision loss: a six-year perspective. J Vis Impair Blind. 2001;95(12):739–48.
2. Senra H, Barbosa F, Ferreira P, Vieira CR, Perrin PB, Rogers H, et al. Psychologic adjustment to irreversible vision loss in adults: A systematic review. Ophthalmology. 2015;122(4):851–61.
3. Binns AM, Bunce C V., Dickinson CM, Harper R, Tudor-Edwards R, Woodhouse M, et al. How effective is low vision service provision? A systematic review. Surv Ophthalmol. 2012 Jan;57(1):34–65.
4. Tabrett DR, Latham K. Adjustment to vision loss in a mixed sample of adults with established visual impairment. Investig Ophthalmol Vis Sci. 2012;53(11):7227–34.
5. Black N. Patient reported outcome measures could help transform healthcare. Br Med J. 2013;346(January):f167.
6. Bruijning JE, van Rens G, Knol D, van Nispen R. Psychometric analyses to Improve the Dutch ICF activity inventory. Optom Vis Sci. 2013;90(8):806–19.
7. Bruijning JE, van Nispen R, Knol D, van Rens G. Low vision rehabilitation plans comparing two intake methods. Optom Vis Sci. 2012;89(2):203–14.
8. Goh D, Subramanian A. Visual hallucinations and eye disease: why Charles Bonnet syndrome is important to eyecare practitioners. Optom Pract. 2012;13(3):127-138.
9. Menon GJ, Rahman I, Menon SJ, Dutton GN. Complex visual hallucinations in the visually impaired. Surv Ophthalmol. 2003;48(1):58–72.
10. Khan JC, Shahid H, Thurlby D a, Yates JRW, Moore AT. Charles Bonnet syndrome in age-related macular degeneration: the nature and frequency of images in subjects with end-stage disease. Ophthalmic Epidemiol. 2008;15(3):202–8.
11. Cox TM, ffytche DH. Negative outcome Charles Bonnet syndrome. Br J Ophthalmol. 2014;98(9):1236–9.
12. Bailie M, Jackson AJ. Diagnosis and management of Charles Bonnet syndrome in a low-vision clinic : a case report. Optom Pract. 2017;18(3):141–4.
13. Bonnet C. L' Essai analytique sur les facultés de l' âme. Copenhagen, C & A Philibert; 1760.
14. Evans JR, Fletcher AE, Wormald RPL, Ng ES-W, Stirling S, Smeeth L, et al. Prevalence of visual impairment in people aged 75 years and older in Britain: results from the MRC trial of assessment and management of older people in the community. Br J Ophthalmol. 2002;86(7):795–800.

15. Quartilho A, Simkiss P, Zekite A, Xing W, Wormald R, Bunce C. Leading causes of certifiable visual loss in England and Wales during the year ending 31 March 2013. Eye. 2016;44(April 2015):1–6.
16. Rumney N. Using visual thresholds to establish low vision performance. Ophthalmic Physiol Opt. 1995;C(1):18-24.
17. Whittaker SG, Lovie-Kitchin JE. Visual requirements for reading. Optom Vis Sci. 1993;70(1):54–65.
18. Carkeet A, Lee L. The slope of the psychometric function for Bailey-Lovie letter charts: defocus effects and implications for modeling letter-by-letter scores. Optom Vis Sci. 2001;
19. Lovie-Kitchin JE. Reading with low vision: The impact of research on clinical management. Clin Exp Optom. 2011;94(2):121–32.

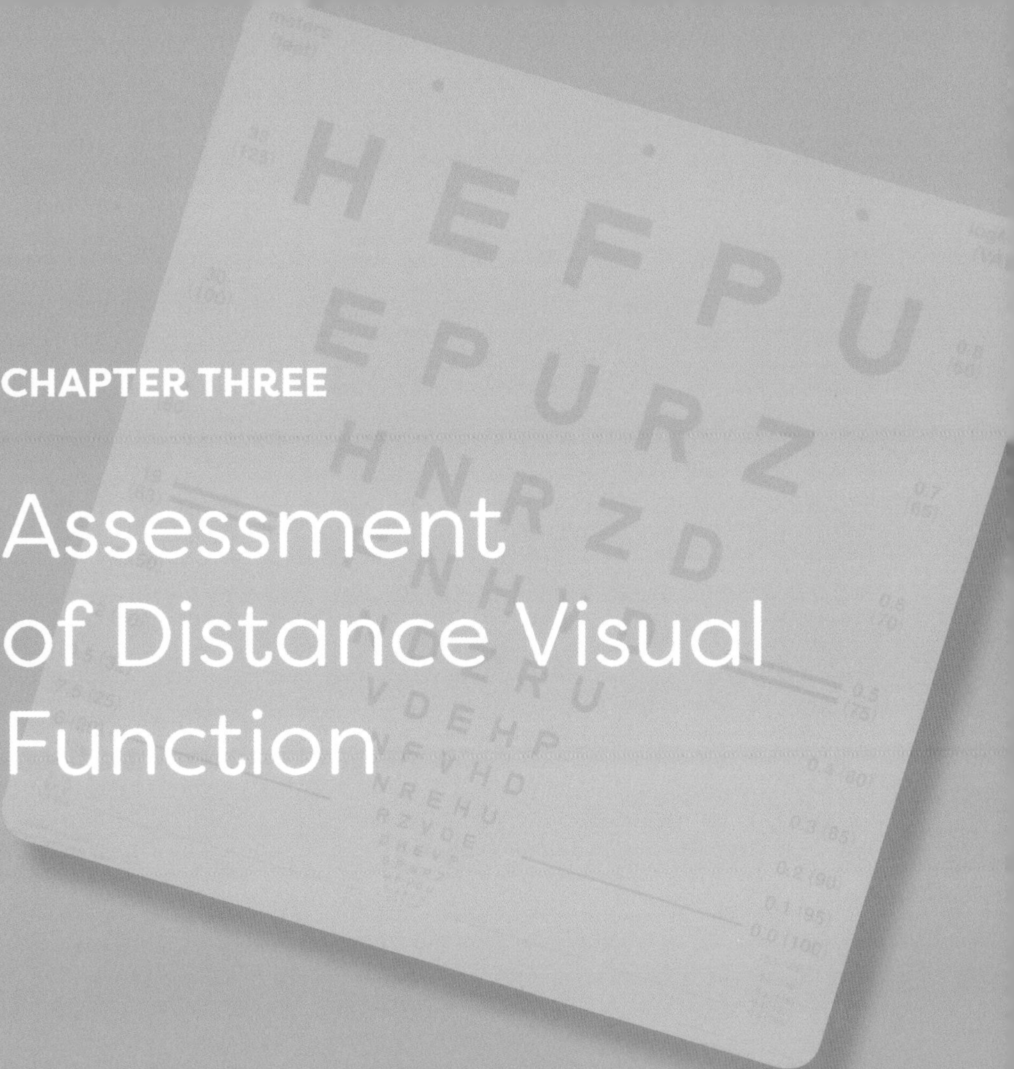

CHAPTER THREE

Assessment of Distance Visual Function

"Our world is not black and white. Good functional vision relies on the ability to see subtle contrast differences. Measurement of contrast sensitivity along with high contrast acuity gives a broader, 'qualitative' understanding of what patients can see. Without this we will not be able to understand the impact of sight loss on activities of daily living."

Dr Louise Gow BSc MSc OD MCOptom, Action for Blind

Assessment of Distance Visual Function

Distance visual acuity

The measurement of distance visual acuity is the most familiar and most widely used test of visual function. However, this is only one in a battery of tests used in the assessment of patients with visual impairment to build a picture of the need and urgency of further treatment, to provide appropriate and timely rehabilitative interventions or to predict the performance of low vision devices.

It follows that our management and prescribing decisions must be made using accurate, reliable and repeatable methods. However, these methods should also be cost effective, easy to administer and as simple to interpret as those tests we use with our normal sighted patients.

The measurement of distance acuity is often the test that many patients with a visual impairment are most anxious about, most assuming that even a small difference from one visit to the next indicates a decline in their eyesight due to changes in their underlying pathological condition. It is also not unusual for low vision patients to have their vision checked by more than one eyecare professional from one appointment to the next. This may also be in a variety of different locations, often using different charts and under different conditions such as lighting or chart distance, etc. Therefore, to be able to answer patients' concerns accurately, measurement of visual acuity must be both **reliable** and **repeatable** so that genuine comparisons may be made between visits. Moreover, if the decision to treat or list for surgery is dependent upon a change in visual acuity, accuracy in acuity measurements is therefore both clinically and financially critical.[1]

Limitations of the Snellen chart

Dutch ophthalmologist Herman Snellen first described the use of single optotypes in the study of vision in the 19th century.[2] Since then, the design of the Snellen chart has changed little over time and still remains today as the most commonly used method of testing and recording of visual acuity in both optometric practice and a large number of hospital eye departments. Furthermore, its use extends into occupational vision standards such as the police and the military, and also other socio-legal documents such as driving licences and visual impairment certification.

However, the limitations of the Snellen chart have been well documented over the years: [3,4]

- When testing patients with low acuity, the chart provides too few letters for a repeatable and consistent visual task
- There is a variable increase in the number of letters on each line, therefore the patient is presented with a task of increasing difficulty
- There is a difference in line legibility between each row, resulting from an inconsistent use of letters with variable legibility
- There is an irregular progression of letter size between lines
- Contour interactions vary throughout the Snellen chart, with the larger letters recording lower acuities having minimal or no crowding effects [5,6]

Despite the weight of evidence that clearly demonstrates the Snellen chart's unreliability, it still remains as the test of choice for a large body of healthcare professionals.

Development of an ideal test chart

Bailey and Lovie successfully addressed the design flaws ingrained within the Snellen chart with the proviso that the measurement of visual acuity should be standardised at all levels on an acuity chart, thus providing an equivalent and repeatable task on each line.[7] To achieve this, only the angular subtense of the letters should change as the patient reads down a chart, with other factors influencing the measurement of visual acuity such as letter spacing or external illumination, ideally remaining exactly the same.

Optotype choice and line legibility

Landolt rings or Tumbling (Illiterate) E optotypes were considered to be the simplest optotype target choices with the Landolt rings chosen as standard in 1909 by the XI International Ophthalmological Congress.[8] One advantage of using this form of optotype is that the resolution task is the same regardless of its orientation. However with only 4 typical presentations, the patient could make a 1 in 4 correct guess.

For each line to have a task of equal difficulty both the number of optotypes per line and the overall legibility of each line should remain constant.[9,10] The move to incorporate letters in a chart provides the practitioner with a test that is easily explained, easy to score, and very quick to administer.[11] Although the use of letter optotypes is a more complex information processing task, the idea of incorporating letters of equal or near equal legibility was attributed first to Woodruff in 1947 and was followed by a more detailed reviewed a few years later in 1965 by Bennett.[12,13] The British Standards Institution consequently recommended the use of 10 non-serifed letters (D E F H N P R U V and Z) presented in a 5x4 grid.[14] This standard has since been updated to include letters C and K with all letters presented on a slightly wider, square 5x5 grid presentation.[15]

The importance of letter legibility was also studied extensively by Sloan who listed a slightly different series of 10 letters (C D H K N O R S V Z) and who also recommended the use of a 5x5 grid presentation.[16]

Scaling and spacing

The size progression of optotypes in a Snellen chart appears arbitrary and does not follow a geometric progression. The concept of using a logarithmic progression of letter optotypes was incorporated into the Keeler A-series charts, developed by Charles Keeler a few years prior to the Bailey-Lovie charts.[17] However, Keeler's focus was to assist the low vision practitioner in establishing a baseline level of magnification rather than an accurate measurement of distance visual acuity.

The Bailey-Lovie charts introduced letter sizing following a logarithmic progression termed logMAR. The term MAR is an acronym for **minimum angle of resolution**, taken as the stroke width of the letter, one fifth of the letter's vertical subtense when printed in the BSI recommended pattern of five stroke widths in height and four stroke widths in width (i.e. a 5 x 4 grid presentation)[14]. LogMAR denotes $\log^{10}$ of the minimum angle of resolution, which in the Bailey-Lovie 6m chart is the logarithm to base 10 of the angular subtense of the optotype stroke width when viewed at 6m. This then creates a logarithmic scale of optotype sizes that decrease in 0.1 logMAR steps.

Between row spacing is equal to the height of the letters in the smaller row and adjacent letter spacing is equal to one letter width. This helps to maintain the same degree of contour interaction throughout the chart.[18]

Standardising external testing conditions

There are several other 'external' factors that also influence the measurement of visual acuity, many of which require review by the practitioner on a regular basis. It is all too easy to forget to re-measure and re-check the calibration of equipment used in the clinic on a regular basis. To ensure repeatability and to maintain consistency between successive visits or to make comparisons between clinic and practitioners, the following factors should also be taken into consideration:

Test distance

Few consulting rooms are 6m in length, which is the testing distance of the original Bailey-Lovie chart. It is often necessary, either due to the constraints of a consulting room or the level of acuity patients present, to move a chart closer than the standard distance. Technically, the clinician may adopt any distance and thus alter the angular size presentation of the letters. However this may make the calculation of acuity scores cumbersome. By moving a logMAR chart closer to the patient in a logarithmic progression, a simple correction factor is added to the overall score.[19] For example, a 6m chart may be moved to 3m and 1.5m and a 4m chart may be moved to 2m and 1m, halving the test working distance each time.

Another reason to alter the test distance is when the patient's acuity is limited to either the top row of letters or the bottom row of letters. As with all charts, the top and bottom rows do not have full contour interaction without having another line either above or below, respectively. Therefore if a patient is unable to read the top line of a chart, then to improve accuracy the chart must be moved closer.

When moving a logMAR chart closer to the patient by half the standard distance, a correction factor of +0.30 logMAR is added to the overall acuity score. Table 3.1 shows the conversion between Snellen and logMAR acuities. Care should be taken when using charts at very close working distances as a small change in head or body posture can make a significant change in the distance between the patient and the chart. This is particularly relevant when testing patients with a central scotoma or media opacities who often move their head and body to catch an eccentric view of the chart.

Table 3.1 Visual Acuity conversion table

LogMAR	6m	20 foot
1.50	6/190	20/632
1.40	6/150	20/500
1.30	6/120	20/400
1.20	6/95	20/320
1.10	6/75	20/250
1.00	6/60	20/200
0.90	6/48	20/160
0.80	6/38	20/125
0.70	6/30	20/100
0.60	6/24	20/80
0.50	6/19	20/63
0.40	6/15	20/50
0.30	6/12	20/40
0.20	6/9.5	20/32
0.10	6/7.5	20/25
0.00	6/6	20/20
-0.10	6/4.8	20/15
-0.20	6/3.8	20/12
-0.30	6/3	20/10

Example:

A 6m Bailey-Lovie chart is placed at 3m and the patient's VA is recorded as +0.60.

The total VA score is 0.60 + 0.30 = 0.90 logMAR (6/48)

Chart luminance

One disadvantage of using externally illuminated and printed charts in a practice or hospital setting is that ambient room illumination tends to be variable from one location to the next. This makes comparisons in values between different clinical settings difficult.

Visual acuity improves with increased chart luminance, until a diminishing rate of increase is reached at the higher luminance levels.[20,21] The luminance level of the test chart is therefore critical in establishing standard test conditions.

Recommended Test Chart Luminance for externally illuminated charts:

- In the UK the recommendation is 120 cd/m^2 [14,15]
- In the US the recommendation is 85 cd/m^2 [9]

However, several studies have concluded that there is not one optimal standard luminance level but rather there is a range of luminance tolerances within which visual acuity testing should be performed. Sheedy suggested a standard luminance level of 160cd/m^2 should be adopted and if a tolerance of +/- 0.02 logMAR acuity were to be acceptable (plus/minus one letter per line in a 5 letter row), then a tolerance range of between 80-320 cd/m^2 would be acceptable. [21]

Methods of scoring

One of the barriers to changing to a logMAR chart has undoubtedly been the need to change to a new method of scoring visual acuity measurements. When assessing Snellen acuity, patients tend to be given credit for a whole line of letters rather than for individual letters seen. With some lines having more letters than others, this method is inconsistent, particularly when fewer letters are available for recording low acuities. Moreover, some Snellen charts do not test acuity beyond 6/6. With no further lines available to record acuities in those patients who are able to see better than 6/6, this truncation in acuity scoring does not represent a true record of the eye's measurement of resolving capability.

Line-by-line termination rule

The most commonly used termination rule is the line-by-line termination rule where the patient is stopped from reading down the chart at the point where they make a set number of mistakes on a line. However there appears to be little agreement over how many mistakes per line should be the termination rule for that chart. A number of practitioners and researchers stop patients reading down a chart when three or more mistakes have been made.[22–24] The patient is asked to complete that line. Carkeet however, argued that there was no rationale in their choice of three in five incorrect letters other than, perhaps clinical experience and went on to explore data modelling to suggest that a termination rule of stopping after four or more mistakes on a line is close to optimum when using Bailey-Lovie or ETDRS eye charts.[25]

Letter-by-letter termination method

Alternatively, a letter-by-letter termination method assumes termination after a certain number of mistakes made over the whole chart with one method allowing the patient to complete the line and another method stopping at the point where a certain number of mistakes have been made. Both methods have been found to have similar results.[25]

Letter-by-letter scoring

Both termination and scoring rules have been shown to have a significant effect on the accuracy of acuity measurements obtained, with methods that assign a visual acuity score in terms of whole lines demonstrating poor repeatability. [22,26–30]

One of the many advantages of logarithmic progression of letter sizing is that it allows for scoring between lines. That is, equal credit is given for every letter read correctly. In the Bailey-Lovie chart, the scale increment between lines is 0.1 logMAR, thus each of the five individual letters may be assigned a score of 0.02. Therefore, if a patient is able to read all of the 0.3 line, plus an additional letter on the next line, he can be given credit for the additional

0.02. His VA score would therefore improve to 0.28. Alternatively, if a patient is only able to read three of the five letters correctly on the 0.4 line, he will have a VA score of 0.44 logMAR.

Example:

- A patient's VA is recorded using a 6m logMAR chart at a distance of 6m
- The patient sees all of the letters on the 0.6 line plus two more from the line below
- VA score calculated as 0.56 logMAR

Example:

- A patient's VA is recorded using a 6m logMAR chart at a distance of 3m
- The patient manages all of the letters on the 0.5 line plus three more from the line below
- VA score calculated as 0.44 + 0.30 to compensate for the 3m working distance = 0.74 logMAR

Example:

- A patient's VA is recorded using a 6m logMAR chart at a distance of 1.5m
- The patient manages to all but one letter on the 0.3 line
- VA score calculated as 0.32 + 0.60 to compensate for the 1.5m working distance = 0.92 logMAR

Using this method of scoring, low visual acuities may be measured and scored as accurately as higher levels of acuity assisting comparison between successive visits. [27,31]

Note: It is still acceptable to additionally record final acuities in equivalent Snellen notation and most logMAR charts will have Snellen acuities printed alongside the logarithmic scale to assist conversion.

Test-retest variability

It is not unusual for practitioners to see fluctuations in visual acuity measurements with no obvious change to the underlying pathology.[22] Test-retest variability (TRV) quantifies this variability in results when the test is repeatedly administered to the same individual even in the absence of true clinical change.

TRV is influenced by a number of factors, including chart design [30] and methods of testing such as termination and scoring rules. There may be significant inter-subject variation due to practitioners varying in their encouragement of the patient, or intra-subject variation as a result of fatigue or personality type where one patient may be more prepared to guess compared to another.[25]

Published values suggest that the TRV of logMAR charts when scored letter by letter for subjects with normal vision requires a change of 0.12-0.18 logMAR to be confident of a clinically significant change in vision.[30,32,33] In comparison, the TRV for a Snellen chart is significantly higher at ±0.33 log units (equivalent to three rows of a logMAR chart) using the more commonly used row-by-row scoring.[32] Additionally, TRV is greater with optical defocus [34] and in patients with age-related macular degeneration.[35]

Whatever the underlying cause of variability, whether it is between patients, practitioners or between same-patient successive visits, the importance is to maintain consistency as far as possible. It is important therefore that practitioners are able to judge the relevance of acuity scores in context, especially when the decision to treat is based upon subtle clinical changes.

Age and shelf-life of charts and reading materials

Plastics and photographic papers used in the production of many charts and tests become grubby over time or degrade with exposure to light. Internally illuminated charts should have their bulbs checked regularly and replaced when required. For example, the the currently available Pelli-Robson contrast sensitivity chart is sold with an expiration date beyond which the chart's accuracy is uncertain.

Distance acuity tests used in the low vision clinic

The Bailey-Lovie Chart

The first logMAR acuity charts were developed by Bailey and Lovie in 1976 and went into production in 1978 (Figure 3.1).[7] The charts are 53x61cm, are externally illuminated and are comprised of a 100% contrast chart on one side and a low 10% contrast chart on the other using the same design principles.

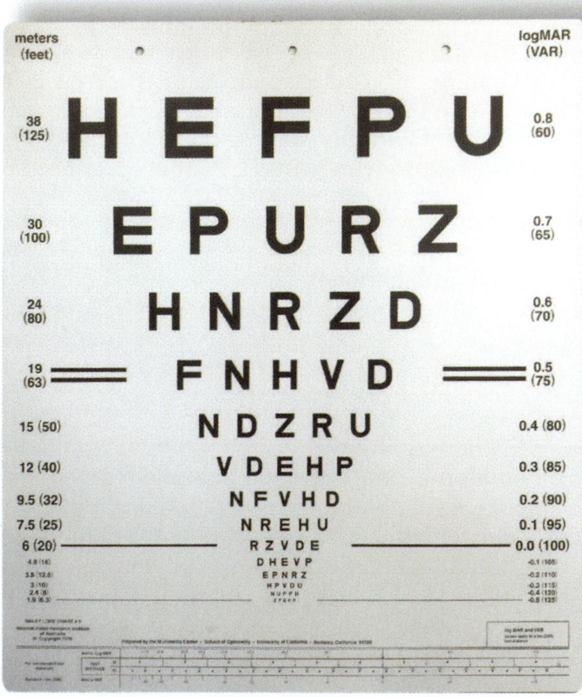

Figure 3.1 Bailey-Lovie charts are 53x61cm with a high contrast chart on one side and a low contrast chart on the other. British standard optotypes are printed in a logMAR progression in a 5 x 4 grid presentation. Recommended luminance for acuity testing is 160 cd/m^2.

The 6m Bailey-Lovie chart has 14 lines of five letters per line, ranging from 0.8 logMAR (equivalent to 6/38) to -0.5 logMAR (equivalent to 6/1.9). Each chart may be scored in Snellen (metric 6m, imperial 20ft) as well as logMAR and VAR (Visual Acuity Rating) scales.

The Bailey-Lovie chart has been shown to provide consistent, accurate and reliable measures of visual acuity with only a small trend for subjects with poorer acuities to improve slightly on a second attempt.[18]

ETDRS Chart

Since the development of the Bailey-Lovie logMAR chart, there has seen the development of several other standardised logMAR charts, all addressing the similar inconsistencies of the original Snellen chart and adopting the design principles outlined by Bailey and Lovie.

Three charts were developed for use in the Early Treatment Diabetic Retinopathy Study (ETDRS),[31] following the same design protocols of the original logMAR acuity test charts. The ETDRS charts (Figure 3.2) consist of sequences of high contrast black letters, silk-screened on a non-reflective translucent washable white polystyrene panel that is usually slotted into a light box containing two fluorescent lamps covered in a reusable fenestrated diffuser sleeve. The charts are therefore internally illuminated.

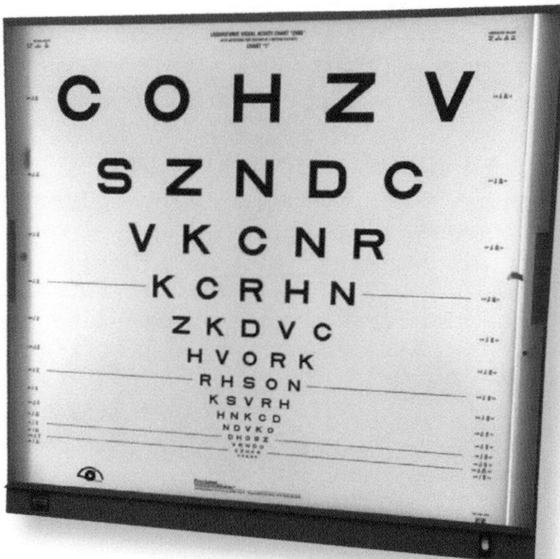

Figure 3.2 The ETDRS charts use Sloan optotypes silk-screened on a non-reflective translucent panel in a 5x5 grid pattern. Charts are slotted into a light box containing two fluorescent lamps. Charts are now available in Llandolt C, Tumbling E and Patti Pics symbols and for use at 4m, 3m and 2m working distances.

The ETDRS chart is designed to be used at 4m, taking this recommendation from the National Research Council Working Group 39[9] due to the then current changes in the US making the charts easier to use in smaller consulting rooms. The original recommendations also suggested the use of ten Sloan letters per line however the charts developed contain five letters per line in a 5x5 grid presentation.

With each Sloan letter assigned with a difficulty score, lines with similar overall difficulty were created for use in Charts 1 and 2 and presented to the R and L eye respectively. Chart R was recommended for refraction of either eye. Following their extensive use in the ETDRS study, the original three charts were revised in 2000, and now incorporate a slight change in the difficulty score for each of the ten Sloan letters used.

The charts are used widely for testing distance visual acuity in both clinical and research settings. Many different types of charts are now available and include Landolt C, Tumbling E and Patti Pics symbols with charts created for use at 4m, 3m and 2m working distances.

The Berkeley Rudimentary Vision Test (BRVT)

The limit of the ETDRS chart is 1.60 logMAR using the chart at the closest recommended working distance of 1m, and for the Bailey-Lovie chart is 1.40 logMAR at 1.5m. For recording lower levels of visual acuity there has not been a widely accepted method with many eyecare professionals still opting to use an unstandardised "Counting Fingers" (CF) or "Hand Movements/Motion" (HM) when the limit of a standard test chart is reached.

However, accurate measurement of severe visual impairment is still important to detect change due to underlying pathology and to consider the need for mobility or rehabilitative services.

The BRVT (Figure 3.3) has been designed to offer a method of testing very low acuity levels.[36,37] Using three sets of cards the BRVT extends the range of acuity to logMAR 2.60 using single tumbling E optotypes, and further to logMAR 2.90 using gratings. Beyond this level, the additional cards of White Field Projection (WFP) and Black White Discrimination (BWD) tests are the last in a battery of thirteen increments that tests from the limit of spatial vision to the perception of light.

Figure 3.3 Using three sets of cards, the BRVT extends the range of acuity from 2.60logMAR using single tumbling-E optotypes to 2.90logMAR using gratings. Beyond this level, the additional cards of White Field Projection (WFP) and Black/White Discrimination (BWD) are the last in a battery of thirteen increments that test from the limit of spatial vision to the perception of light.

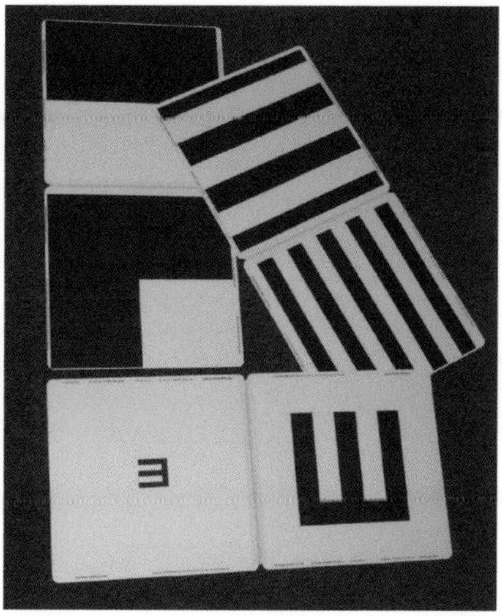

The Moorfields Acuity Chart

Using the design principles incorporated into the ETDRS chart, the Moorfields Acuity Chart (MAC) (Figure 3.4) uses 'vanishing' optotypes.

'Vanishing' optotypes are of high-pass design (low spatial frequencies removed) and are constructed with a black core and white edges with the mean luminance equal to the grey background that they are printed on. Known as high-pass filtered letters,[38] they are unlike conventional optotypes; the letters have near identical detection and resolution thresholds under foveal viewing conditions in normal subjects and thus appear to 'vanish' at the point their resolution threshold has been reached.

Visual acuity measurements with the vanishing optotypes are less affected by termination rules and scoring methods[39] and the use of vanishing optotypes has been shown to reduce the TRV inherent in logMAR charts in patients with uncorrected refractive error.

One study suggested that the MAC is also more sensitive in detecting functional loss in patients with AMD compared to conventional letter chart designs such as the ETDRS with similar TRV [40] which may have implications in the earlier detection of the disease.

Ideally, a logMAR distance chart should be used to assess all patients with low vision. Both the ETDRS and Bailey-Lovie charts are ideal for this purpose and have similar repeatability. Together with the BRVT, an accurate assessment of all levels of distance vision may be quickly scored

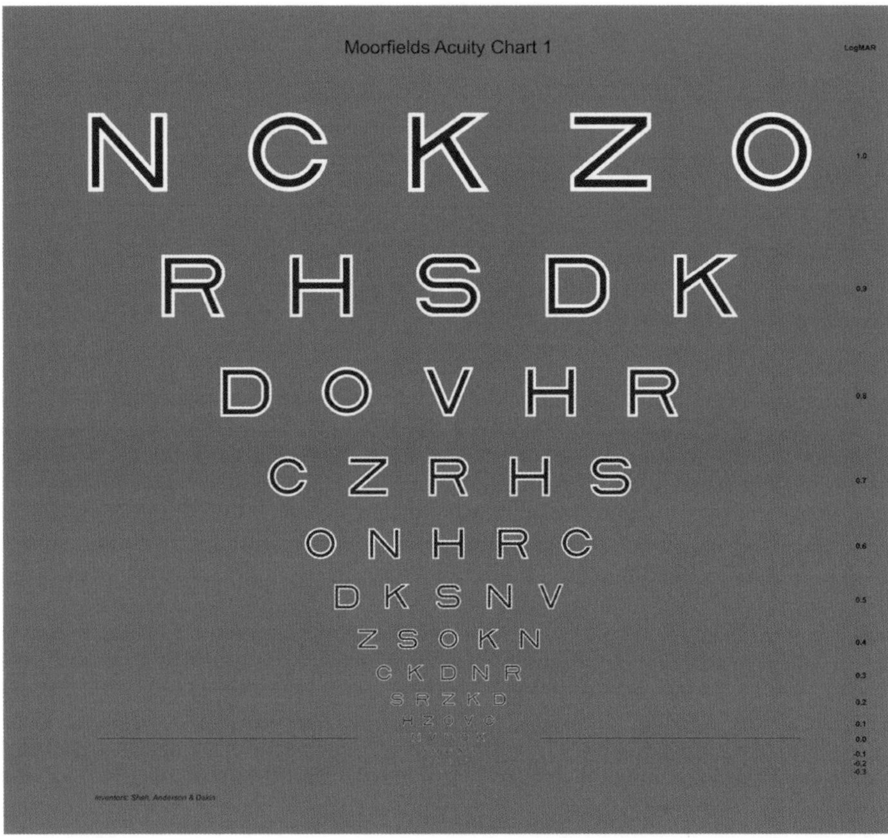

Figure 3.4 The Moorfields Acuity Chart.
Image courtesy of developers Nilpa Shah, Roger Anderson & Steven Dakin (www.moorfields.nhs.uk)

in logMAR with a simple conversion to the more familiar Snellen equivalent if still preferred. The ETDRS has the advantage over the Bailey-Lovie in maintaining consistent illumination, however the light box into which the test cards are slotted is large and may take up space in a small consulting room. The Bailey-Lovie takes up little space although may be slightly more difficult to achieve even illumination.

Contrast sensitivity

The measurement of contrast sensitivity (CS) has been a well-established test used in clinical and research settings to assist diagnosis and progression of pathological conditions.[11] In the low vision setting, patients who have significantly reduced contrast sensitivity function report difficulties discerning kerbs and steps, which have implications on the patient's mobility and susceptibility to falls. [41]

Contrast sensitivity is also a significant predictor of self-reported activity limitations in daily living tasks,[42] including reading.[43]

Pelli-Robson letter contrast sensitivity chart

Sloan letters are printed in sixteen triplets of letters with each triplet having the same level of contrast. The contrast of each triplet progressively reduces by 0.15 logCS log units as the patient reads down the chart, while the size of the letters remains the same (Figure 3.5). [11]

The original recommended near addition of +0.75DS to compensate for the 1m working distance has since been shown to have no significant influence on results,[44] therefore patients need only wear their habitual distance correction. Participants are encouraged to read until no letters in a given triplet are read correctly, allowing for a viewing time of at least 15-20 seconds when close to contrast threshold.[45]

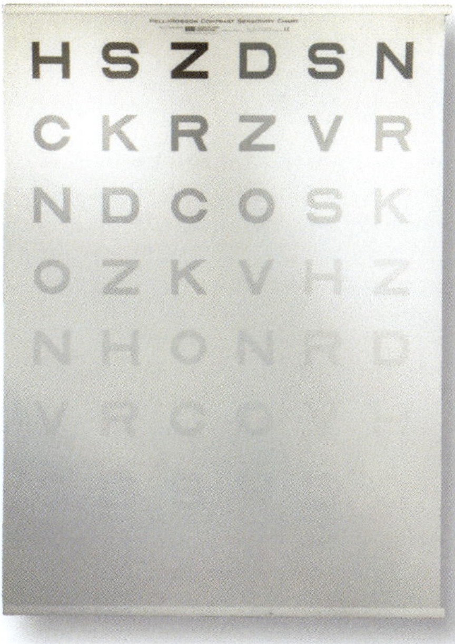

Figure 3.5 Pelli-Robson contrast sensitivity chart is 59cm wide and 84cm high is viewed at 1m with a recommended luminance of 85 cd/m^2. Each letter subtends 2.8° at the recommended viewing distance of 1m, which is above acuity threshold for most low vision patients.

Contrast sensitivity is scored by giving credit of 0.05 logCS unit for each individual letter read correctly after the first triplet.[46,47] Results can be described as representing severe, significant, or noticeable loss, or normal contrast sensitivity (Table 3.2).

Table 3.2 Percentage and logCS values for the Pelli-Robson chart

Loss of contrast sensitivity	Pelli-Robson letter triplet	Contrast	logCS	Pelli-Robson letter triplet	Contrast	logCS
Severe	VRS	99%	0.0	KDR	63%	0.15
	NHC	44%	0.30	SOK	31%	0.45
Significant	SCN	22%	0.60	OZV	15%	0.75
	CNH	11%	0.90	ZOK	7.8%	1.05
Noticeable	NOD	5.6%	1.20	VHR	3.9%	1.35
	CDN	2.8%	1.50	ZSV	1.9%	1.65
Normal	KCH	1.4%	1.80	ODK	1.0%	1.95
	RSZ	0.7%	2.10	HVR	0.5%	2.25

Mars letter contrast sensitivity test

Whilst the Pelli-Robson chart is widely used in research it has been less well received in clinical practice, requiring a large wall space with even illumination that may be difficult to obtain in some consulting rooms. The Mars test (Figure 3.6) is portable, easier to store and easier to illuminate evenly. It uses the same set of Sloan letters but contrast declines by letter in 0.04 logCS unit steps.

With similar design principles, the Pelli-Robson and Mars charts have been shown to have similar Test-retest variability (TRV) of ±0.21 and ±0.20 log units respectively for both normal and low vision patients.[48] Normally sighted patients under 50 years of age will have a contrast sensitivity score of 1.80 logCS or better, dropping to 1.65logCS in the older age group.

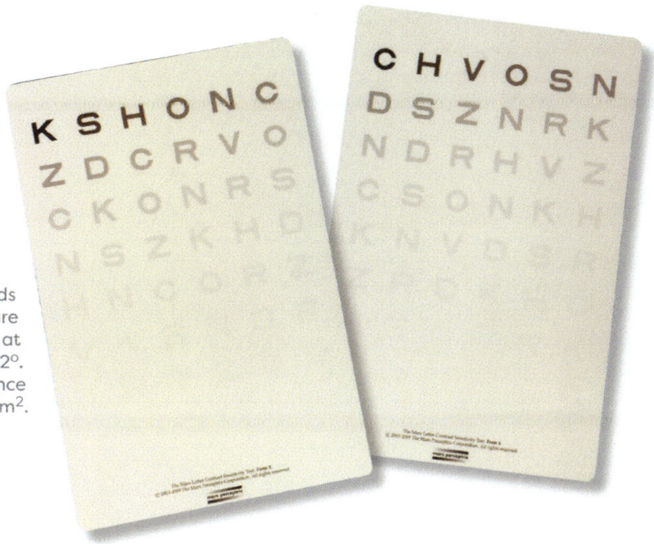

Figure 3.6 The Mars cards are 22.8 x 35.6cm and are intended for use at 50cm at which each letter subtends 2°. recommendation luminance is 85cd/m².

Visual field assessment

The assessment of the visual field on those with low vision, especially with central vision loss can be difficult and is often largely overlooked by many low vision practitioners. However, the consequences of visual field loss have functional implications with the ability to perform many daily living activities and with mobility. For example, a right hemianopic defect will have a significant impact upon reading from left to right. A left hemianopic defect has an impact upon the reader navigating back to the beginning of the next line in a block of text. An inferior visual defect will have an impact upon seeing food on a plate and all defects, both central and peripheral, can result in reduced orientation and mobility and an increased risk of falls or fear of falling.[49,50] Visual field loss is therefore a significant factor influencing activity limitations in patients with visual impairment.[51]

Clinical assessment of visual fields is usually completed monocularly and is used largely in the detection and monitoring of disease progression. However, an assessment of the binocular visual field is more useful to the low vision practitioner as most tasks of daily living are completed with both eyes open.[52] Both central (0-30°) and peripheral (30-60°) binocular visual fields should ideally be assessed; although both areas of the visual field have been shown to have an impact upon patients' functional ability, with most impact as a result of peripheral field loss.[49]

Electronic charts, apps and downloads

Computerised charts have been in use in optometry practice and hospital clinics since the 1990's. With the advancement of technology to produce high-resolution images the large array of tests includes logMAR and contrast sensitivity charts. For use in a low vision setting, the same design principles as

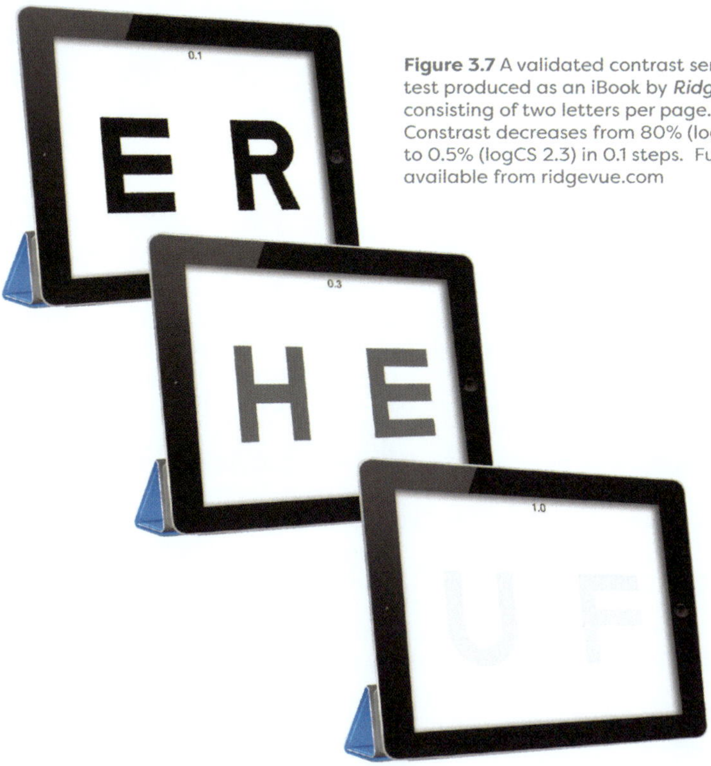

Figure 3.7 A validated contrast sensitivity test produced as an iBook by *Ridgevue* consisting of two letters per page. Constrast decreases from 80% (logCS 0.1) to 0.5% (logCS 2.3) in 0.1 steps. Full details available from ridgevue.com

previously discussed must be met, together with appropriate validation and must conform to the relevant agreed standards.

The advantages of using electronic systems with low vision patients include the presentation of larger character sizes, randomisation of character or word presentation and automatic scoring. There is no image degradation over time and the portability of using a laptop or tablet favours use over the larger cardboard charts, which are less portable, and which degrade over time. Care however must be taken when using smaller screens, which may not allow for appropriate control of contour interaction when presenting large targets and control of calibration is required, especially when producing a chart to measure contrast sensitivity (Figure 3.7).

References

1. Reeves B, Hill A, Aspinall P. The clinical significance of change. Ophthalmic Physiol Opt. 1987;7(4):441–6.
2. Snellen H. Test-types for the determination of the acuteness of vision. 1862.
3. Lovie-Kitchin JE. Is it time to confine Snellen charts to the annals of history? Ophthalmic Physiol Opt. 2015;35(6):631–6.
4. Elliott DB. The good (logMAR), the bad (Snellen) and the ugly (BCVA, number of letters read) of visual acuity measurement. Ophthalmic Physiol Opt. 2016;36:355–8.
5. Flom M, Heath GG, Takahashi E. Contour interaction and visual resolution: contralateral effects. Science. 1963;142(3594):979–80.
6. McGraw P, Whitaker D, Winn B. Reliability of the Snellen chart. Br Med J. 1995;310:1481–2.
7. Bailey I, Lovie-Kitchin JE. New design principles for visual acuity charts. Am J Optom Physiol Opt. 1976;53(11):740–5.
8. Nordenson J. Ophthalmic International Standards, 1950. Br J Ophthalmol. 1951.
9. National Research Council. Recommended stardard procedures for the clinical measurement and specification of visual acuity. Report of working group 39. Adv Ophthalmol. 1980 Jan;41:103–48.
10. Sloan L, Rowland W, Altman A. Comparison of three types of test target for the measurement of visual acuity. Q Rev Ophthalmol. 1952;8:4-15.

11. Pelli D, Robson J. The design of a new letter chart for measuring contrast sensitivity. Clin Vis Sci. 1988;2(3):187–99.
12. Woodruff E. Visual acuity and the selection of test letters. Some recent advances. Ophthalmic Opt Trans London Hatt Press. 1948;59–70.
13. Bennett AG. Ophthalmic test types. A review of previous work and discussions on some controversial questions. Br J Physiol Opt. 1965 Jan;22(4):238–71.
14. BSI 4274-1. British Standard Specifcation for test charts for determining distance visual acuity. Br Stand Inst. 1968;BS 4274-1.
15. BSI 4274-1. Visual Acuity Test Types- Part 1: Test charts for clinical determination of distance visual acuity - Specification. 2003 p. 1–10.
16. Sloan L. New test charts for the measurement of visual acuity at far and near distances. Am J Ophthalmol. 1959;48:807–13.
17. Keeler C. Visual aids for the pathological eye; excluding contact lenses. Trans Ophthalmol Soc United Kingdom. 1956;76:605–14.
18. Lovie-Kitchin JE. Validity and reliability of visual acuity measurements. Ophthalmic Physiol Opt. 1988;8(4):363–70.
19. Bailey I, Lovie-Kitchin JE. The design and use of a new near vision chart. Am J Optom Physiol Opt. 1980;57(6):378–87.
20. Hecht S. The relation between visual acuity and illumination. J Gen Physiol. 1928;11:255–81.
21. Sheedy JE, Bailey I, Raasch T. Visual acuity and chart luminance. Am J Optom Physiol Opt. 1984;61(9):595–600.
22. Raasch T, Bailey I, Bullimore MA. Repeatability of visual acuity measurement. Optom Vis Sci. 1998;75(5):342–8.
23. Brown B, Lovie-Kitchin JE. Repeated visual acuity measurement: establishing the patient's own criterion for change. Optom Vis Sci. 1993;70(1)45-53.
24. Lovie-Kitchin JE, Brown B. Repeatability and intercorrelations of standard vision tests as a function of age. Optom Vis Sci. 2000;77(8):412–20.
25. Carkeet A. Modeling logMAR visual acuity scores: Effects of termination rules and alternative forced-choice options. Optom Vis Sci. 2001;78(7):529–38.
26. Ferris F, Bailey I. Standardising the measurement of visual acuity for clinical research studies. Ophthalmology. 1996;103(1):181–2.
27. Bailey I, Bullimore M, Raasch T, Taylor H. Clinical grading and the effects of scaling. Investig Ophthalmol Vis Sci. 1991;32(2):422–32.
28. Arditi A, Cagenello R. On the statistical reliability of letter-chart visual acuity measurements. Investig Ophthalmol Vis Sci. 1993;34(1):120–9.

29. Vanden Bosch ME, Wall M. Visual acuity scored by the letter-by-letter or probit methods has lower retest variability than the line assignment method. Eye. 1997;11:411–7.
30. Hazel C, Elliott DB. The dependency of LogMAR visual acuity measurement on chart design and scoring rule. Optom Vis Sci. 2002;79(12):788–92.
31. Ferris F, Kassoff A, Bresnick G, Bailey I. New visual acuity charts for clinical research. Am J Ophthalmol. 1982;94(1)91-96.
32. Rosser D, Laidlaw D, Murdoch I. The development of a "reduced logMAR" visual acuity chart for use in routine clinical practice. Br J Ophthalmol. 2001;85:432–6.
33. Lim L, Frost N, Powell R, Hewson P. Comparison of the ETDRS logMAR, "compact reduced logMar" and Snellen charts in routine clinical practice. Eye. 2010;24:673–7.
34. Rosser D, Murdoch I, Cousens S. The effect of optical defocus on the test–retest variability of visual acuity measurements. Invest Ophthalmol Vis Sci. 2004;45(4):1076–9.
35. Patel PJ, Chen FK, Rubin GS, Tufail A. Intersession repeatability of visual acuity scores in age-related macular degeneration. Investig Ophthalmol Vis Sci. 2008;49(10):4347–52.
36. Bailey I, Jackson a. J, Minto H, Greer RB, Chu M a., Sturrock BA, et al. The Berkeley Rudimentary Vision Test. Optom Vis Sci. 2012;89(9):1257–64.
37. Bailey IIL, Lovie-Kitchin JE. Visual acuity testing. From the laboratory to the clinic. Vision Res. 2013;90:2–9.
38. Howland B, Ginsburg A, Campbell F. High-pass spatial frequency letters as clinical optotypes. Vision Res. 1978;18(8):1063–6.
39. Shah N, Dakin S, Whitaker H. Effect of scoring and termination rules on test-retest variability of a novel high-pass letter acuity chart. Invest Ophthalmol Vis Sci. 2014;55:1386–92.
40. Shah N, Dakin SC, Dobinson S, Tufail A, Egan CA, Anderson RS. Visual acuity loss in patients with age-related macular degeneration measured using a novel high-pass letter chart. Br J Ophthalmol. 2016;0:1–7.
41. Morrison-Fokken A, Dunne M. Falls risk assessment in optometric practice: an introduction to non-visual and visual risk factors. Optom Pract. 2014;15(2):39–48.
42. Tabrett DR, Latham K. Factors influencing self-reported vision-related activity limitation in the visually impaired. Investig Ophthalmol Vis Sci. 2011;52(8):5293–302.
43. Latham K, Tabrett DR. Guidelines for predicting performance with low vision aids. Optom Vis Sci. 2012;89(9):1316–26.
44. Latham K, Hughes JA. Is a reading addition necessary for clinical contrast sensitivity measurements? Poster presentation EAOO, Malaga, April 2013. 2013.

45. Elliott DB, Sanderson K, Conkey A. The reliability of the Pelli-Robson contrast sensitivity chart. Ophthalmic Physiol Opt. 1990 Jan;10(1):21–4.

46. Elliott DB, Whitaker D, Bonette L. Differences in the legibility of letters at contrast threshold using the Pelli-Robson chart. Ophthalmic Physiol Opt. 1990;10:323–6.

47. Elliott DB, Bullimore MA, Bailey I. Improving the reliability of the Pelli-Robson contrast sensitivity test. Clin Vis Sci. 1991;6(6):471–5.

48. Dougherty B, Flom R, Bullimore M. An evaluation of the Mars letter contrast sensitivity test. Optom Vis Sci. 2005;82(11):970–5.

49. Subhi H, Latham K, Myint J, Crossland MD. Functional visual fields: relationship of visual field areas to self-reported function. Ophthalmic Physiol Opt. 2017;37(4):399–408.

50. Ivers RQ, Cumming RG, Mitchell P, Attebo K. Visual impairment and falls in older adults: the Blue Mountains Eye Study. J Am Geriatr Soc. 1998;46(1):58–64.

51. Tabrett DR, Latham K. Factors influencing self-reported vision-related activity limitation in the visually impaired. Investig Ophthalmol Vis Sci. 2011;52(8):5293–302.

52. Asaoka R, Crabb DP, Yamashita T, Russell RA, Wang YX, Garway-Heath DF. Patients have two eyes!: Binocular versus better eye visual field indices. Investig Ophthalmol Vis Sci. 2011;52(9):7007–11.

CHAPTER FOUR

Refracting Patients with a Visual Impairment

“Provision of an up-to-date refractive correction and good lighting for a patient with low vision has the potential to minimise the magnification required in low vision aids, or in some cases to reduce the need for additional devices.”

Dr Keziah Latham BSc PhD FCOptom Prof Cert LV FHEA
Anglia Ruskin University, Cambridge, UK.

Refracting Patients with a Visual Impairment

Introduction

Following a detailed task analysis and assessment of distance visual function (Chapters 2 and 3) some practitioners will opt to include a refractive assessment before prescribing low vision aids or magnification. Whether completed by themselves or by another practitioner, this chapter outlines some of the considerations that may be relevant when refracting patients with a visual impairment.

Patients with progressive sight loss often find visual assessment stressful and occasionally distressing, especially when they have become aware of a further reduction in visual function. It is not uncommon for the patient to be anxious and, therefore, it is worth taking the time to make them comfortable and to allow as much time as possible. A patient who is stressed may not perform as well as they can and, therefore, the accuracy of the assessment could be compromised.

However, refracting patients with low vision is often quicker and less complicated than for patients with 'normal' acuity. For example, the number of check tests that can be done is significantly fewer.

Adapting the assessment

Measuring Visual Performance

Methods of recording distance and near visual performance are covered in more detail in Chapters 3 and 5. However, it is essential to be as accurate as possible. Practitioners should remain cautious when comparing results between visits due to the number of factors that influence Test-Retest Variability (TRV). A drop in visual acuity due to poor repeatability can easily be misinterpreted as a further loss due to ongoing pathology. Secondly, the relationship between distance and near acuities and subsequent magnification calculations will be much easier if there is an accurate starting point. For example, neither the use of 'counting fingers' (CF) nor '<6/60' give a useful measurement of vision/visual acuity (V/VA).

For ultra-low vision, practitioners may opt to use the Berkeley Rudimentary Vision Test (Figure 3.3, Chapter 3). Only use hand movements (HM) or light perception (PL) when the vision is just that. A V/VA of HM or less has no functional vision and will not improve with magnification devices. Patients with this level of acuity may need further referral or signposting for sensory assistance.

A V/VA of, for example 3/60 (1.30 logMAR) however, may benefit with the very high-powered LVAs for limited survival reading.

Using a phoropter

Basic refraction equipment is all that is necessary to examine patients with a visual impairment. A suitable trial frame or Halberg clip is preferred to a phoropter head. Patient's with central scotoma or distortion or who have hazy, patchy media may move their head around to eccentrically view the targets presented. Nystagmus patients may also prefer to adopt an abnormal head posture (AHP) at which point their amplitude of nystagmus is in check.

The phoropter has the disadvantage of reducing the light levels that may influence the low vision patient's visual performance. It also prevents the practitioner from observing facial expressions, something of great use to an experienced practitioner.

Qualitative assessment of central acuity

Allow time for patients to describe what they can and cannot see and make a note within their record card. For example, patients with hemianopia will report letters missing within the field loss, and patients with central vision loss will describe missing letters, areas of patchy vision or distortion. It is useful to note whether the patient is using eccentric viewing during vision assessment. For example, if they describe that they can see the end letters when looking at a central letter, the patient may benefit from encouragement to exploit this eccentric viewing ability (Chapter 10).

Contrast sensitivity and glare

Many low vision practitioners will measure contrast sensitivity (Chapter 3). A reduction in contrast sensitivity should immediately highlight the need to incorporate advice about orientation and mobility, the use of contrast or colour contrast within the home, or whether a full home lighting assessment may be beneficial (Chapter 10). A reduction in contrast sensitivity also has a bearing on prescribing low vision devices[1] (Chapter 5). Some practitioners may opt to take V/VA measurements using an external glare source such as a pen-torch or a Brightness Acuity Test (BAT) and to determine influence upon acuity. Such an approach is simple and often very effective at simulating the detrimental effect glare may have on a patient's vision.

Cover test

A cover test is useful to establish the primary fixating eye. Use large targets, whatever is appropriate to the level of vision. The measurement taken will be gross. A previously amblyopic or squinting eye, which now retains the better acuity, will not necessarily be the primary fixating eye. The patient may still use the eye with the lower acuity, particularly if there has been a long-standing squint. This will have implications when prescribing magnification or monocular units.

An eye with an acquired defect and low vision may become divergent with time. This is often seen in those patients who have been referred for cataract surgery several years after the eye has become divergent. In such cases, intractable diplopia may occur.

Use larger steps

A patient with an acuity of, for example, 3/60 (1.30 logMAR) will not be able to appreciate a difference of ±0.25. Therefore, use steps appropriate for the level of V/VA. For example, start by using ±1.00 spheres, then reduce to ±0.75 and so on until the patient is unable to discriminate the difference.

Cross-cylinders

In addition to the usual equipment for refraction, cross-cylinder lenses of ±0.75, ±1.00 and ±1.50DC are available. ±0.25 sphere and cyl changes have limited value on any low vision patient with an acuity of less than approximately 6/24 (0.60 logMAR). It is important to remember that with lower levels of visual acuity, the ability to discriminate between two blurred presentations becomes increasingly difficult. Added to this, a patient with a central scotoma may have a variable acuity during a subjective routine. Thus, the need for obtaining an accurate endpoint must always be balanced with a realistic view of the reliability of the patient's subjective responses.

Refract at a closer working distance

LogMAR charts have the advantage of being able to be presented at any distance, as discussed in Chapter 3. For example, a 6m Bailey-Lovie chart may be used at 3m and 1.5m. The original 4m ETDRS charts may also be presented at 2m and 1m. ETDRS charts 1 and 2 are recommended for use with the R and L eyes respectively, and chart R is recommended for refraction of either eye.

If the test chart and object of regard are set closer than 6m, then the refraction result obtained might not be accurate for viewing a target in the far distance. This will have a bearing on the final prescription:

Example:

An eye that is looking at an object at 2m will need an adjustment of 0.50D to the final prescription, i.e. if the patient was found to have a prescription of +1.75D at 2m, then the final distance refraction will be adjusted to +1.25D.

Arguably, this small difference will have little impact on a patient with poor visual acuity. As acuity reduces it is often found that the patient looks into the distance rarely and objects within arm's length become more important. Similarly, it is not uncommon for some practitioners to consider leaving the patient overcorrected for a closer television viewing distance or viewing a CCTV for example at very close distances. Caution must be exercised if deliberately over-correcting the patient in their distance spectacles when this may have an impact upon their peripheral vision and mobility.

Larger refractive errors and cylindrical corrections

Many patients have stopped wearing spectacles as they offer little subjective difference. However when prescribing magnification, significant refractive errors should still be corrected to enhance the image where possible. Therefore it is important for patient to bring any old spectacles along to the assessment.

Correction of a significant refractive error or sizeable cylindrical correction may improve peripheral image quality and has implications on mobility. An accurate distance or near spectacle prescription may be essential when using a fixed-focus stand magnifier, or mounting a telescopic unit. Refer to Chapters 6 and 8 for further detail.

Pinhole

Macular problems often show significantly reduced VA when using a pinhole. Corneal problems that improve significantly with a pinhole, may justify a contact lens trial. On rare occasions, where the primary cause of impairment is a loss of media clarity, (such as corneal, vitreous or lens disease), there may be a visual improvement with a pinhole that may not be achievable with corrective lenses or optical appliances. This may leave the patient frustrated or unhappy with the aids prescribed.

Record near working distance

It is fundamental to record all near working distances accurately when working with patients with a visual impairment. Quite often a patient will be adopting a working distance close to or within the focal length of the plus lens magnifier. The patient may find the working distance acceptable for low-powered plus lenses; however the lens-object working distance of a high-powered plus lens will be significantly shorter. For example, maximum magnification of a +10.00D lens will be achieved with a working distance of 10cm.

An uncorrected -4D myope will have a working distance of approximately 25cm, equivalent to his/her far point. Similarly, a -10D myope may have found an unaided vision of N5 when holding text at a 10cm working distance. This is similar to a patient using a +10D spectacle magnifier. Encouraging the -10D myopic patient to adopt the close working distance may be all that is necessary for him rather than prescribing an expensive, complicated device.

Domiciliary visits

The advantage of a domiciliary visit is the ability to assess the patient within their own environment instead of a brightly lit clinical environment of an eyecare practitioner's consulting room. Many older patients are reluctant to modify their home environment. For those who have ultra-low vision, a significant alteration to their familiar setting requires adaptation and therefore the home-based assessment and advice given should include discussion on how prepared the patient is to incorporate any changes. For those with early dementia, significant modifications should be approached with caution as these can be distressing. Whilst sitting closer to the television may be the best advice and provided with all good intentions, most older patients are not keen to make a change to the layout of a room, especially if they are living with a spouse or family member who may also be affected by the change. In such circumstances, an 'occasional chair' that may be pulled out for convenient short spells in front of the television may be more acceptable.

Adaptations made for specific eye conditions

Nystagmus

Congenital nystagmus is one of the most common causes of visual impairment in children. It may occur without any other evidence of ocular associations (idiopathic), or it may occur in association with another congenital condition such as albinism or rod monochromatism.

The amplitude of nystagmus and thus the patient's V/VA may drop with stress, fatigue or high illumination levels. Patients with nystagmus often demonstrate a significant reduction in monocular acuities when one eye is occluded during refraction.

The amplitude of the nystagmus may reduce with convergence when reading or when adopting an abnormal head posture (AHP) to achieve a 'null-point.' The null-point is the point at which the nystagmus is dampened, the visual acuity optimal, and thus the point at which the patient will have optimal discrimination during refraction. Therefore, allow the patient to adopt whatever AHP they feel is most comfortable. Make a note in the record card or take a photograph; an AHP may have implications on what type of low vision aid to demonstrate. It is also an excellent reason to avoid using a phoropter as previously mentioned.

Therefore, it follows that if the amplitude of the nystagmus increases significantly during refraction, then it is likely that an accurate refractive endpoint will be more difficult to achieve. The practitioner must try to manage the nystagmus so that the patient may achieve maximum discrimination.

In summary

- Avoid full occlusion by using fogging techniques to refract the patient binocularly. The patient is more likely to demonstrate better acuity with both eyes open than with one eye occluded.
- Allow the patient to adopt their AHP, even if this appears quite extreme. By allowing the patient to attain his/her null-point, the nystagmus may be dampened to a degree where the pendular movements are checked and the VA achieved is at its maximum.
- Patients who present with roughly equal V/VA in each eye, and due to the dampening of the nystagmus, will often prefer binocular devices despite having poor or absent binocular function (Chapters 8, 11).
- Patients often demonstrate a better near visual acuity than what would have been expected from their distance visual acuity. Convergence for a near target may dampen the nystagmus significantly. This may have implications on the strength or device prescribed.

Albinism

There are two major types of albinism (total oculocutaneous and ocular), and the visual acuity varies between them. A patient with albinism may present with astigmatic errors, squint, photophobia and nystagmus. Due to abnormal decussation of the chiasmal nerve fibres, patients with albinism do not demonstrate true binocular function.

All refractive errors should be fully corrected especially in children as often the full hypermetropic correction, if present, can significantly reduce or eliminate the need for near aids. Nearly all children with albinism can achieve N12-N8 or better with simple refractive correction. By accommodating, the children merely hold the reading material close to gain the necessary 'magnification' effect; the associated convergence may also dampen their nystagmus.

Patients with albinism are truly photophobic due to the reduction or complete lack of pigment within the eye. A tint will always be needed out of doors with additional UV protection. However, if glare sources are managed appropriately, then patients often prefer normal or near normal task illumination.

During refraction, those who are severely photosensitive may benefit from reducing the background room illumination slightly or turning off the illumination from within an internally illuminated test chart. However, when recording V/VA, standardised chart lighting must be maintained.

Children with nystagmus are further discussed in Chapter 11.

Congenital cataracts

Early diagnosis of congenital cataract is vital. All new-born children should ideally be checked for a clear ophthalmoscopy reflex within the first few days of life.

If there has been early surgical intervention there may be a chance of binocular function. Frequent refraction is then very important since the level of hypermetropia drops quite rapidly as the eye develops during the first few years of life. With a clear retinoscopy reflex and no accommodative effort, objective refraction can be accurate; a satisfactory endpoint is readily achieved with even the smallest of children by working directly on axis. However, a severe uniocular cataract imposes difficult management, with a uniocular contact lens offering the best possible solution.

Many children with aphakia are fitted with contact lenses from an early age when possible. For the majority, a reading addition of +4.00 to +6.00D addition is usually adequate, as they will naturally have working distances shorter than those of adults. For those children wearing full spectacle correction, a 30% larger image size also has its advantages.

Communication

The importance of a relaxed environment and the time to listen cannot be overemphasised. The longer one works in visual impairment, the more one realises that much of the benefit for the patient is gained from having a knowledgeable and empathetic person listen to them and discuss their visual condition with them.

No two patients are alike; for one individual the activity limitations may be overwhelming and will have an substantial impact upon their emotional health, while for another, personal coping strategies may lessen the impact on their lifestyle and quality of life. Patients with congenital eye disorders learn to adapt from an early age whereas loss of sight in adult life may be more challenging. Adjustment to acquired vision loss is complex[2] and it is worth remembering that one device which works well for one patient may not be acceptable to another.

The fact that many patients learn most about their eye disease from the internet is a sad reflection of the fact that no eyecare professional has taken the time to fully explain the underlying condition. Most patients can cope better with their impairment if they understand it. The eyecare practitioner is ideally placed to give this sort of information and a few minutes spent explaining the condition is often invaluable. Much of this time is often spent dispelling various myths as patients arrive with a whole variety of misunderstandings which can affect their motivation and ability to adapt.

Chapter 12 discusses the impact and adjustment to vision loss in more detail.

Motivation

A patient's motivation will influence the management approach. Poor motivation may be part of the coping strategy of the patient or a defence mechanism and if they genuinely feel they cannot carry out a task such as reading then it would be unwise to push them. The most effective approach is to be reassuring without being forceful or prescriptive.

Simple goal-setting within a realistic timescale is central; a careful choice of an achievable task might be the starting point that the patient needs. Continued observation and contact time between patient and practitioner are also useful for building confidence which in turn will improve motivation.

Summary

- The practitioner needs to be sensitive to the patient's emotional response to their impairment, especially so in the case of an acquired impairment. A patient with age-related macular degeneration may present having had 70 years' worth of good functional vision that has been lost over the last few months. In many cases, the first appointment may deal primarily with advice and counselling to allow for some acceptance and rationalisation of the situation before any care plan is embarked upon.
- The absence of external signs of the problem, combined with the general perception that blindness means total lack of visual function, often implies that relatives and carers of the patient are less supportive than might be expected. Simulation spectacles may be helpful in this context (Figure 4.1)
- By setting realistic and achievable goals is a simple yet effective way of increasing patient involvement in their care plan.

References

1. Latham K, Tabrett DR. Guidelines for predicting performance with low vision aids. Optom Vis Sci. 2012;89(9):1316–26.
2. Tabrett DR, Latham K. Adjustment to vision loss in a mixed sample of adults with established visual impairment. Investig Ophthalmol Vis Sci. 2012;53(11):7227–34.

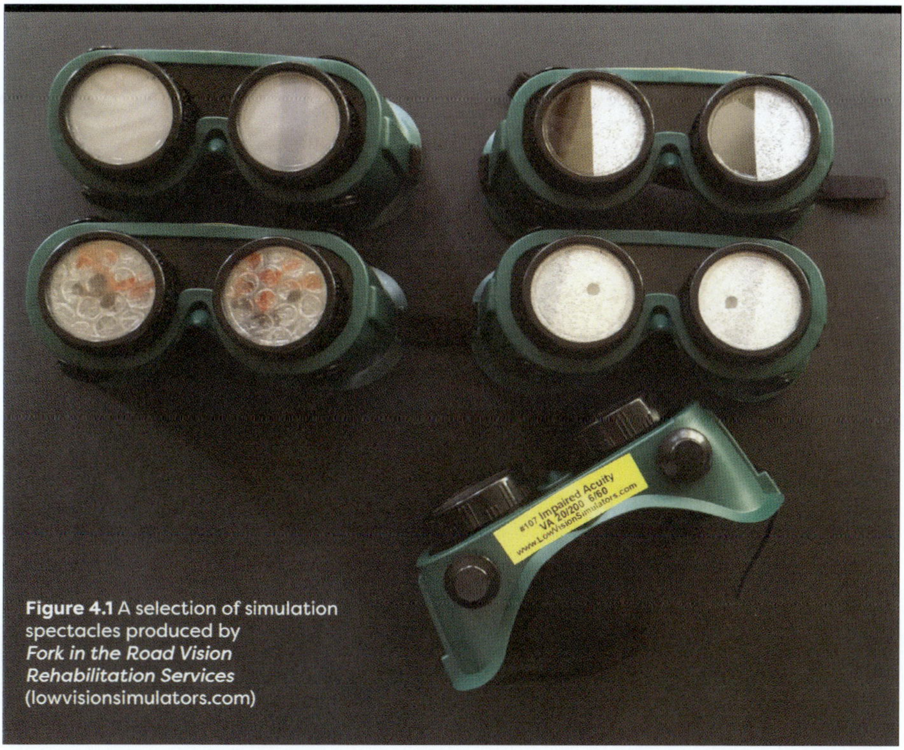

Figure 4.1 A selection of simulation spectacles produced by *Fork in the Road Vision Rehabilitation Services* (lowvisionsimulators.com)

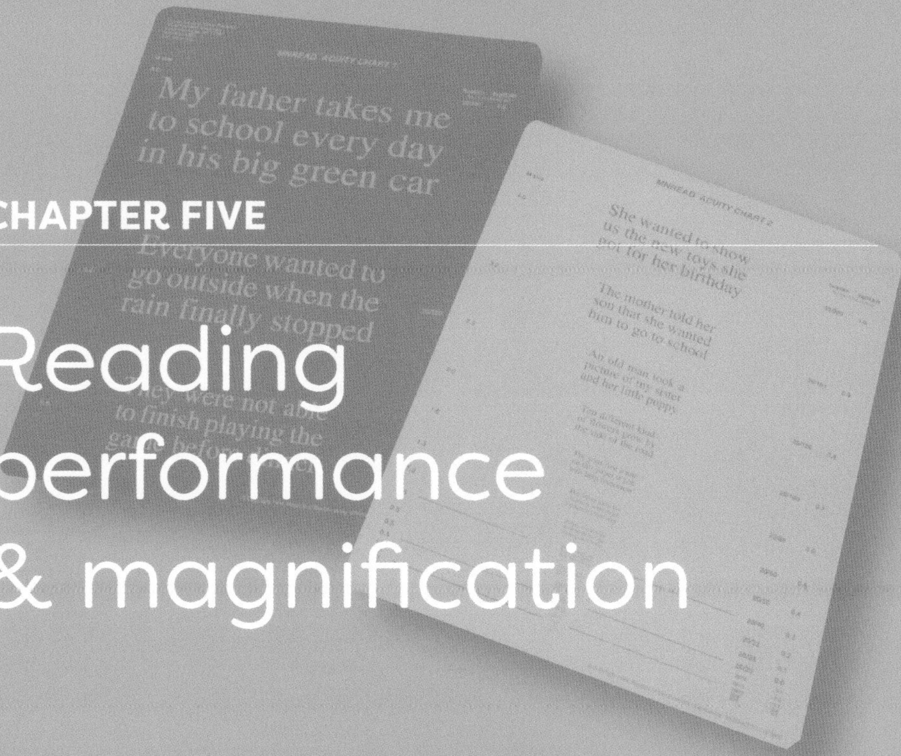

CHAPTER FIVE

Reading performance & magnification

> "When examining patients that have low vision it is important to adopt a holistic approach. This is even more crucial when working with older people or those who have special needs. It involves a high level of communication, not only with the patient and immediate family, but also all those involved in the well-being of the patient."

Dr Zahra Jessa PhD BSc MCOptom

Moorfields Eye Hospital and Royal National Institute of Blind People, London, UK

Reading performance & magnification

Introduction

For the majority of patients with low vision, reading is their most important goal,[1,2] with many daily living tasks relying on the need to see small physical print sizes of varying degrees of colour, contrast and quality.

Although distance and near acuities are related, they are not equivalent. Reading is also a more complex task involving accurate eye movements and higher cognitive aspects of comprehension.[3–5] Thus, a multifaceted assessment is required to set realistic and achievable goals for an individual with low vision.

During assessment, patients should be encouraged to read to their limit of resolution to ensure threshold is reached. Working distances should always be measured as this determines the retinal image size of the print being viewed and has implications on calculating the level of magnification needed when prescribing low vision devices.

However, practitioners should be mindful that there may be a significant difference between what patients can push themselves to read and what they subjectively consider as comfortable. Thus, assessment of an individual's reading performance and making a judgement on the required magnification for various tasks is based upon many factors. Whilst this chapter outlines the theory of magnification and addresses some core rules for addressing task magnification such as the need for acuity reserve, how a patient uses a low vision device varies considerably between one individual and another. Variations in the effect of magnification are caused by how the device is used, from the power of the patient's habitual prescription, to how far the magnifier is held away from both the eye and the page.

Angular print size or physical print size?

LogMAR near acuity

Angular print size refers to the angular subtense of print on the retina and is recorded in logMAR. Angular print size takes into consideration both the physical print size and the working distance at which the print is held. Therefore, the working distance at which the chart is held is always recorded, for example 0.9 logMAR at 40cm.

The physical print size is a description of the actual size of the printed text on the page and therefore remains unchanged regardless of working distance. The physical print size is more functionally relevant to the patient whose goal may be to read a specific size of text such as newsprint. Physical print sizes include the familiar N point notation or Sloan M units.

N point

N point notation is based upon typographic measurements where a Point is a printer's measure of 0.0139 inch (0.353mm). There is a linear relations ship between the print sizes: N5 is half the size of N10; N18 is three times larger than N6, etc.

Sloan M

The M unit designates the distance (in metres) at which the object subtends 5' arc.[6,7] Bailey et al measured 1M to be equivalent to N8-N9[8,9] although Latham and Tabrett found that the physical print size of the 1M print size incorporated into the MNREAD charts is slightly larger than N10.[10] The relationship between the two print sizes is not exact. Table 5.1 shows a conversion chart to assist practitioners in understanding the comparable relationship between physical print size and angular print size.

Table 5.1 Conversion chart for near acuity

Angular print size		Comparable physical print sizes	
LogMAR at 25cm	LogMAR at 40cm	N Point	Closest equivalent Sloan M Unit
1.7	1.5	100	
1.6	1.4	80	10
1.5	1.3	64	8.0
1.4	1.2	48	6.3
1.3	1.1	40	5.0
1.2	1.0	32	4.0
1.1	0.9	25	3.2
1.0	0.8	20	2.5
0.9	0.7	16	2.0
0.8	0.6	12	1.6
0.7	0.5	10	1.3
0.6	0.4	8	1
0.5	0.3	6	0.8
0.4	0.2	5	0.63
0.3	0.1	4	0.5
0.2	0.0	3	0.4
0.1	-0.1	2.5	0.32
0.0	-0.2	2	0.25
-0.1	-0.3	1	0.20
-0.2	-0.4		0.16
-0.3	-0.5		0.13

Example: a physical print size of N8 is equivalent to an angular print size of 0.4 logMAR when the print is held at 40cm, or 0.6 logMAR when held at 25cm.

Near acuity tests used for low vision assessment

There is a wide variety of near vision test charts available. Most offer high contrast blocks of N point text ranging from N48 to N5 or N4.5. Charts are available in a number of fonts but most tend to use Times New Roman as it is one of the most widely used typefaces still used in general printing. While an accurate measurement of near acuity is arguably required for comparisons between successive visits, many patients comment that the high contrast of a printed test card bears less resemblance to the ability to read at home. The large majority of tasks that patients seek to read will vary in colour and contrast which may degrade with age or continued use over time.

The Bailey-Lovie word reading chart

The Bailey-Lovie near charts (Figure 5.1) are constructed of a similar logarithmic design to their distance counterparts. The use of unrelated words rather than sentences removes contextual cues that influence fluency and which may overestimate reading acuity.[8] The charts present a wider range of print sizes from N80 to N2 (10M to 0.25M in Sloan M units) and in a logarithmic progression from 1.6 to 0.0 logMAR when held at 25cm.

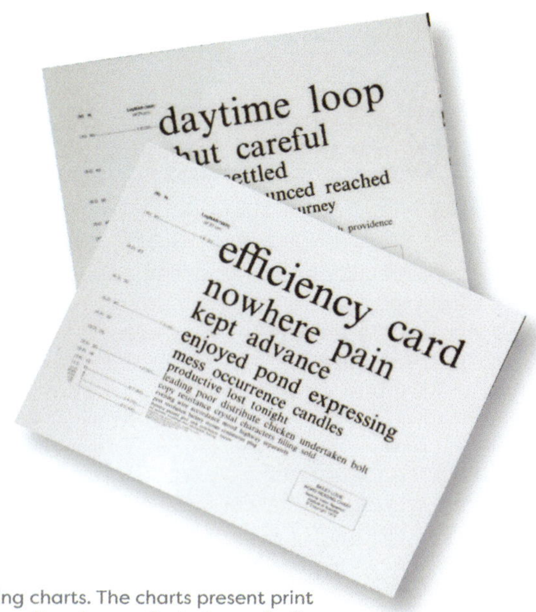

Figure 5.1 The Bailey-Lovie word reading charts. The charts present print size from N80 to N2 and are printed in Times New Roman font, chosen for its widespread use in most newspapers and books

The MNREAD near acuity charts

The Minnesota low vision-reading chart[11,12] (Figure 5.2) is a continuous text reading chart, using short single sentences printed onto 3 lines with the level of difficulty standardised by using the same number of characters in each sentence (60 characters, 10 standard length words). The cards are printed in high contrast, and print size reduces in 0.1 log steps from logMAR 1.3 to -0.5 (N64 to N1; 8M to 0.13M) when used at the recommended working distance of 40cm (with appropriate correction if required). Charts are also available in reverse contrast print. Recommended chart luminance is a minimum of 80 cd/m^2.

As with a distance logMAR chart, MNREAD charts can be used at shorter working distances to extend the range of angular acuity that may be assessed.[13] Changes to the appropriate near correction may be required from the +2.50D addition used at 40cm. For example, if the patient is unable to read at the recommended working distance of 40cm using a +2.50D reading addition where appropriate, the chart can be moved to half the distance, i.e. a working distance of 20cm and a reading addition of +5.00D may be required. The logMAR near acuity is adjusted by adding 0.3 logMAR to the final score (Chapter 3).

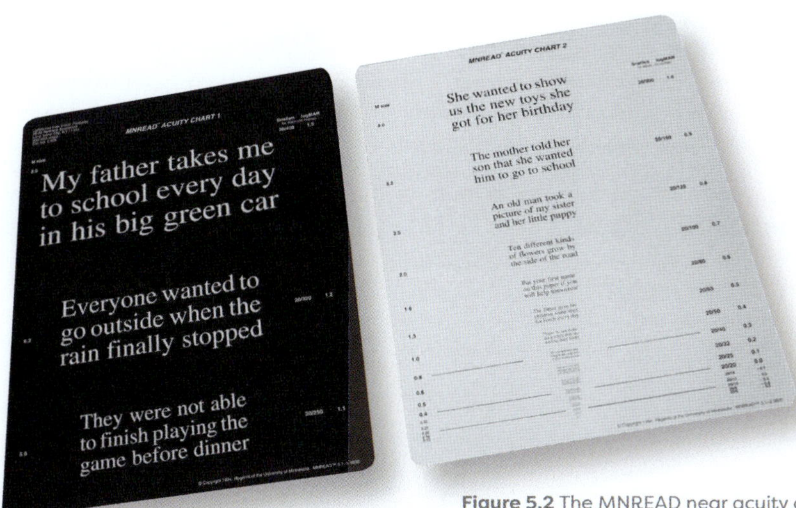

Figure 5.2 The MNREAD near acuity charts in standard and reverse contrast print

The MNREAD charts have been found to have a test-retest variability (TRV, Chapter 3) of ±0.05 logMAR for reading acuity in normally sighted subjects and a higher value of ±0.10 logMAR in patients with low vision.[14,15] TRV values for the Bailey-Lovie word reading chart in normal subjects are ±0.10 logMAR.[16]

The Maclure Reading Test

When assessing children with low vision, it is important to be able to assess a child's ability to see to read rather than their ability to read. The Maclure Reading Test contains reading material of varying difficulty or standards appropriate for different age groups. It has been designed specifically for use with children and is therefore not specific for use in low vision. However, one disadvantage is that the child's age group appears at the top of the printed text, and this can be off-putting for those children who are sensitive to their reading capabilities or for those with special needs. Assessment of children and young people is discussed further in Chapter 11.

Factors affecting reading performance

Reading rate

Reading rate rather than near acuity has been shown to be a more relevant outcome measure when assessing low vision patients with a view to prescribing magnification.[17] Reading rates vary between patients as a consequence of individual reading abilities, however a minimum reading rate of 80-100 words per minute (wpm) is considered to be an appropriate guideline for fluent reading, whereas for more brief tasks or spot reading the reading rate ideally should be 40 wpm or more.[18,19] Reading speeds can be determined quickly and efficiently using the MNREAD near acuity charts.[20]

Acuity and contrast reserves

A number of visual factors are known to influence reading performance in patients with low vision, specifically acuity and contrast reserves, the number of characters visible within the field of view and the scotoma size, where relevant.[4,18] The most significant of these factors is acuity reserve, described as the ratio between the print size of the task to the patient's acuity threshold (near reading acuity). When considering acuity reserve in the context of reading rates, the critical print size (CPS) is the smallest print size that supports reading at the patient's maximum reading speed (MRS).[21]

In practical terms, having some acuity in reserve means that the patient is not working on the limit of vision when viewing a task. The complexity of the task determines how much acuity reserve is needed:

- Spot task or survival reading, e.g. cooker dial, a calendar entry
- Sustained or fluent reading tasks e.g. reading a column of newsprint

In other words, viewing a near task on or close to the limit of vision is possible (such as looking at a cooker dial) but sustaining this whilst reading a column of newspaper print over a period of time may be more of a struggle to achieve. Therefore, for sustained reading, more magnification will be required to maintain some acuity in reserve.

Contrast sensitivity is often significantly reduced in patients with low visual acuity; if a task involves poor quality print, simply making the task or object larger will not improve its visibility. Therefore, it follows that a level of contrast sensitivity in reserve is also required to improve both spot and sustained reading tasks. Chapter 3 outlines methods for assessing a patient's contrast sensitivity in a practical setting.

Current recommended values are listed below: [4,18,22,23]

Spot Reading Tasks

- Estimated reading speed of 40 (wpm)
- An acuity reserve of 1.3:1 (task print size: patient's acuity threshold)
- Equivalent to 0.1 log unit or 1 line of a near logMAR chart
- Contrast reserve of 3:1
- Field of view (no. characters visible) 1

Fluent Reading Tasks

- Estimated reading speed of ≥100wpm
- A minimum acuity reserve of 2:1
- Equivalent to 0.3 log units or 3 lines on a near logMAR chart
- Contrast reserve of 10:1
- Field of view (no. characters visible) 4-6

If a patient needs to be able to read a column of newsprint successfully (N8 approximately), then we need to prescribe sufficient magnification for her to be able to read at least N4 or better. (Reserve of acuity 2:1). If the patient is given an aid with which she can only achieve N8, then it is less likely that reading newsprint will be sustained for any length of time.

Note: when considering these guidelines, the commonly used Faculty of Ophthalmologists Times New Roman Chart does not have a range of print sizes great enough for use with low vision patients. Many patients may not be able to see the largest print size of N36 or N48. Furthermore, to measure reserves of near acuity, especially when the patient is using a magnification device, the chart may need to present very small print sizes, such as those found in the Bailey-Lovie word reading chart (Figure 5.1).

Some worked examples are listed below:

Spot reading task e.g. reading kitchen scales

A patient manages N24 with best-corrected spectacles. She would like to be able to see her digital kitchen scales whilst measuring ingredients for a cake. The size of the task is estimated as N18. Working on the principle that she needs a **1.3:1** reserve of acuity to see this spot reading task, she requires sufficient magnification in a device to achieve N18 / 1.3 = N14 (approx.). N24 to N14 is approximately 1.7x magnification.

Sustained reading task e.g. reading a telephone directory

A patient manages N18 with his current glasses. He would like a magnifier to be able to find a number in a telephone directory. The print size of the directory is approximately N6. Working on the principle of needing a reserve of acuity of **2:1** for a sustained viewing task, he needs a magnifier that will allow him to achieve a print size of N3 (N6/N3 = 2:1 reserve). Therefore, to improve his near VA from N18 with his current glasses to N3, the patient would need approximately 6x magnification (N18/N3).

To achieve spot reading task of 40 wpm or a fluent reading speed of ≥100 wpm, the guidelines suggest a contrast reserve of 3× and 10× respectively.[4,18] Therefore, printed text of 80% contrast could be predicted to be fluently read by someone with 8% contrast threshold (1.05 logCS, boundary of significant/noticeable loss), or spot read by someone with 30% contrast threshold (0.45 logCS, boundary of severe/significant loss) (Table 3.2, Chapter 3).

In a study by Latham and Tabrett,[10] it was established: for patients whose near acuity is worse than 0.85 logMAR at 40 cm and whose goal is to read 1M(N8) with a low vision device, if their contrast threshold is better than 1.05logCS (i.e. half way down a Pelli-Robson chart), then 1M is should be achievable with a low vision aid and that the patient is likely to achieve a fluent reading rate. If worse than 1.05 logCS, then 1M print is less likely to be accessible, even with low vision aids.

Although this model is not completely predictive,[10] it serves as a useful guide as to whether or not the practitioner should discuss alternative options other than optical magnification to achieve the patient's personal goals, such as the use of electronic devices offering contrast enhancement or sensory substitution methods such as audio books.

Methods of estimating task magnification

When choosing a magnification device for a patient there are a number of methods that may be used to estimate the strength needed to view the task comfortably, taking any reserves into consideration. It must be noted however that the methods used, either theoretical or practical are merely an estimate but they do serve to give the practitioner a starting point with which to base an assessment of task magnification. How well individuals perform with a magnification device depends upon a number of other clinical and psychological factors.

Using near acuity charts

All near charts described may be used to estimate task magnification. The relationship between lines of N point notation was discussed in the previous section. In summary, magnification between N point sizes is a simple ratio. For example, N20 is twice as large as N10 and four times as large as N5.

The magnification between each line of all logMAR charts, distance and near, is 1.26x. Thus, for every 3 lines of change (0.3 log units) there is a 2x difference in magnification. In other words, magnification between lines of a logMAR chart is calculated as a product of each line difference and not as the number of lines difference: e.g. 3 lines difference is calculated as 1.26 x 1.26 x 1.26 = 2.00 x (Table 5.2).

Table 5.2 Magnification factor between the number of successive lines of logMAR acuity

Lines of improvement in logMAR	Magnification required
1	1.26x
2	1.6x
3	2x
4	2.5x
5	3.2x
6	4x
7	5x
8	6.4x
9	8x
10	10x

Example:

A patient manages N40 on a Bailey-Lovie word reading chart at a working distance of 40cms (thus 1.1 logMAR or 5M). Her aim is to read through a ready-meal catalogue for planning her next order. The task size is N10. Taking into consideration that she needs a reserve of acuity for this sustained viewing task, we should aim to give her a magnifier with which she should be able to see N5 (N10:N5 = 2:1 reserve).

Magnification required may be calculated in three ways:

- She will require x8 magnification to improve her current near acuity from N40 to N5 (N40/N5 = 8x).
- Alternatively, the magnification difference in lines of logMAR is 9 lines: from 1.1 logMAR to 0.2logMAR (Table 5.2) and thus 8x.
- Similarly, the difference between Sloan 5M to 0.63M is also 8x. (5M/0.63M = 7.93x).

Example:

If a patient has an acuity threshold of N32 (4M) and their goal is to read N8 fluently with an acuity reserve of 2:1, then the aim would be to provide sufficient magnification to achieve N4 comfortably (i.e. N8:N4 = 2:1 reserve). Theoretically, the magnification required to achieve this would be 8x (N32/N4).

Example:

If a patient has an acuity threshold of 0.6 logMAR at 40cm (1.6M) and their goal is to spot read a task of size 0.4 logMAR (1M), then the aim would be to provide sufficient magnification to achieve the line below this to provide some acuity reserve (0.30 logMAR at 40cm, 0.8M). An improvement of 0.3 logMAR, or 3 lines, is therefore required, and, the magnification theoretically required to achieve this would be 2x (1.6M/0.8M=2x).

Practical assessment of task magnification

Quite often patients' expected near acuity or performance with the estimated task magnification is unexpected or spurious. This may be down to a number of factors, such as the nature of the underlying pathology. Patients with ARMD, for example, will often demonstrate a significantly reduced near acuity than expected due to the presence of a central scotoma or distortion. Posterior subcapsular cataracts can also give anomalous results; the cataract is close to the nodal point of the eye and despite relatively good distance acuity, the near VA can be quite poor in comparison. Furthermore, pupillary constriction may enhance the influence of scotomata and opacities in one individual, whilst it may give an improvement in vision similar to a 'pinhole' effect in another.

Similarly, macular distortion may also record a significantly worse near acuity than expected. Patients with nystagmus, however, may achieve better acuity at near due to the dampening of their nystagmus upon convergence at closer working distances.

The methodical step-by-step routine outlined below is an extremely useful method of estimating task magnification and more representative in outcome terms than using the charts, as with every additional step increase in lens power, both patient and practitioner can see the effect of magnification on the text in view. Furthermore, by increasing the lens power gradually, the shorter working distances, reduction in field of view and the importance of lighting can be demonstrated:

- Establish the patient's distance prescription.
- Establish the patient's baseline near acuity with a +4.00D addition at the focal length of 25cm ('unit' magnification, x1). Note the near acuity achieved.
- Increase the near addition power presented at near until the desired acuity is met. This is usually done in +4.00D steps. Encourage the patient to bring the object or text into the focal length of the new equivalent lens power.

  E.g. +8.00D addition, the new working distance will be 12.5cm
- For each increase in near addition, note the acuity and the working distance.
- When the desired near visual acuity is met, the magnification of the near addition thus demonstrated gives the practitioner a starting point magnification with which to demonstrate the device of choice, such as a hand magnifier i.e. start with a magnifier with similar equivalent lens power.

The 'divide-by-three' rule

This 'rule' has been previously used to estimate near acuity based on the distance Snellen acuity using equivalent triangles and dividing the denominator of the Snellen acuity by a factor of three. For example, for a distance acuity of 6/24, the predicted near acuity would be 24÷3=N8 at a working distance of 25cm (assuming any relevant near correction in place). This method is only approximate and should be used in context with an understanding of its limitations. For example, posterior subcapsular cataracts, where the opacity is closer to the nodal point of the eye may result in a significantly reduced near visual acuity compared to that recorded in the distance.

Methods of magnification and M=F/4

Methods of magnification can often appear complicated but in practical terms it is simply the comparison between two different sized images. How those images are resized will vary according to the technique used, such as moving in closer to an object, or physically enlarging it. For example, if we cannot see the number plate of a car, we walk up closer to it. Similarly, we regularly advise our patients to sit closer to the television if they are struggling to see it. If we struggle to see small print on our computer screen or tablet, we can simply make it bigger. All are methods of magnification that increase the angular subtense of the object at the eye and thus the size of the retinal image.

Thus, magnification can be described as the ratio of the angle of subtense at the retina of an object to the increased angle when it is magnified.

Relative distance magnification

If the patient moves in towards a television by half the total distance, (for example from 3m to 1.5m), then the television will appear twice as large.

$$\text{Magnification} = \frac{\text{Old object distance}}{\text{New object distance}} = \frac{3\text{m}}{1.5\text{m}} = \times 2$$

This is termed relative distance (approach) magnification and is the basis of the optical magnification employed in our hand, stand and spectacle magnifiers.

To be able to make comparisons more consistent between visits, between individuals or between practitioners, we need an agreed reference point when discussing near magnification. This reference point is our 'old object distance' and by convention is set at 25cm. This is also often termed as 'the least distance of distinct vision', as for most of us, convergence is still possible at this distance so it represents a sensible baseline distance on which to assess near visual function.

For example, if a patient needed to bring the print in to 12.5cm in order for it to be seen, then the retinal image size is 2× larger than it would be if it had been held at 25cm, our agreed conventional starting point:

$$M = \frac{25\text{cm}}{12.5\text{cm}} = \times 2$$

From this equation comparing old and new object distances, and on the assumption that 25cm is the conventional 'old' object distance, we derive the magnification formula, M = F/4. Alternatively, if we chose a conventional starting point of 50cm, the resultant magnification formula would be M = F/2.

What the lenses do is to merely focus the retinal image of the object at the given distance, in this case a +4.00D addition for a 25cm working distance, and a +8.00D addition for a 12.5cm working distance. Alternatively, the patient may wish to use their accommodative effort, if they have it. Thus, it is typical for a child with a visual impairment to hold text very close in order to achieve 'magnification' of the print or object. Myopes may remove their spectacles to achieve a similar effect.

Therefore, taking 25cm as our reference point as unit (x1) magnification:

+4.00D at 25 cm	1×
+8.00D at 12 cm	2×
+10.00D at 10 cm	2.5×
+20.00D at 5 cm	5×

From this, we can describe a +4.00D lens as having unit magnification. Each successive increase of another 4 dioptres adds another unit of magnification. It is important, however to remember magnification is relative, a ratio comparing old and new object distances. From the patient's point of view, the magnification they will achieve with any low vision device will be based on the comparison of what they can now see with the new device compared to their habitual situation.

Labelling of low vision devices: nominal vs. trade magnification

If one assumes an object Q to be placed at the anterior focal plane of the lens before an emmetropic eye E, then the image formed Q' will be formed at infinity (Figure. 5.3). If one then looks at the situation before the lens was in place (Figure 5.4) then the magnification M will be the ratio of the two angles of subtense, u'/u. The two angles may be defined in terms of the triangles they are within, such that u = −h/p and u' = −h/f. If the values are now put in to replace the angles in M = u'/u, then one is left with M = −pF. If one then assumes p to be −25cm (sometimes termed the 'least distance of distinct vision') then one is left with the formula:

$$M = F/4$$

This is called the **nominal magnification formula**, but is based on several assumptions as outlined and also does not really represent how an aid might be used. More typically, an object will be held within the anterior focal plane of the lens such that an image is formed closer than infinity (Figure 5.5). If one now assumes that the object is placed close enough so that the image is formed at the anterior focal plane of the lens, say −25cm for consistency, then algebraic derivation based on Figure 5.4 will lead to the formula:

$$M = F/4 + 1$$

In order to arrive at this, the value d representing the lens-to-eye distance must be assumed to be zero and the image-to-eye distance q must equal p in the unaided eye (which is −25 cm). This so-called **trade magnification formula** is the one some manufacturers still subscribe to. However, it often differs significantly from the actual magnification a patient will achieve when using the low vision device.

Other methods of magnification used in low vision practice to increase the size of the retinal image are:

Relative size magnification

Can be defined as the increase in an angle of subtense resulting from making something physically larger.

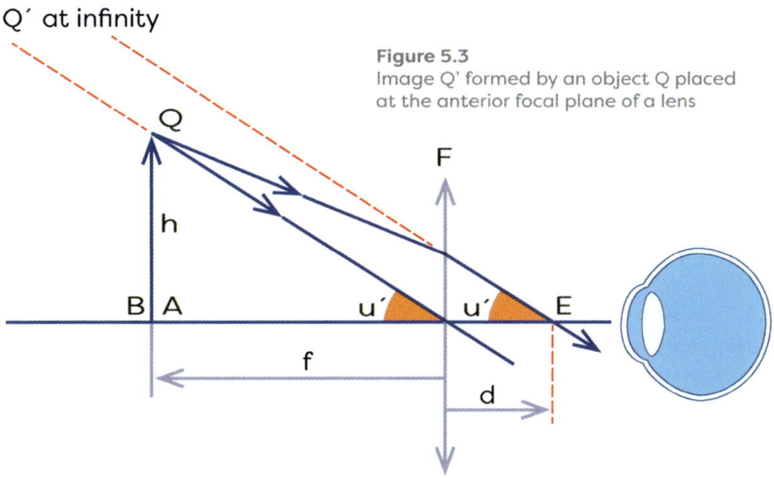

Figure 5.3
Image Q' formed by an object Q placed at the anterior focal plane of a lens

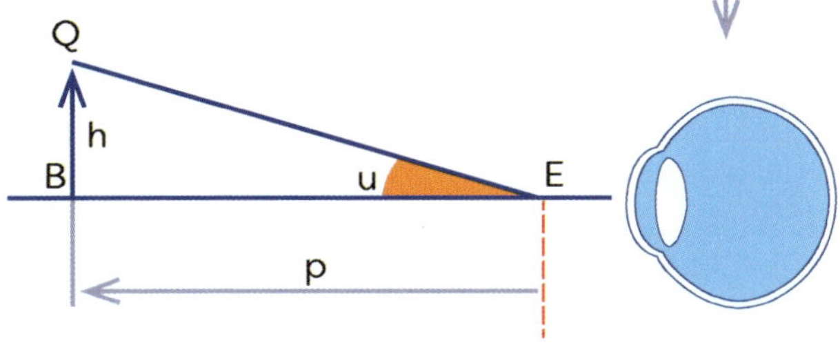

Figure 5.4
Situation before the lens was in place

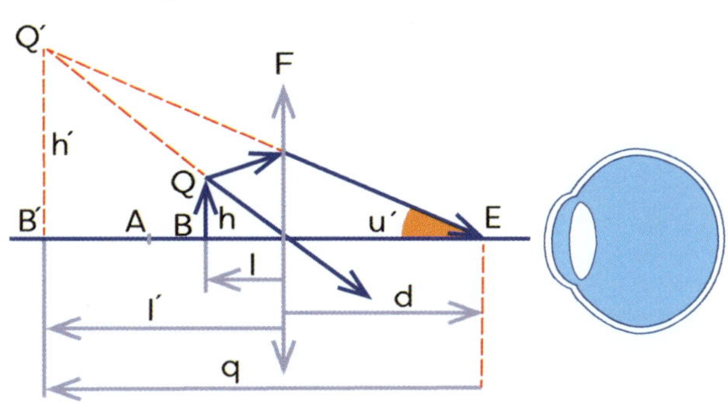

Figure 5.5
Image Q' formed closer than infinity

object Q, image Q', eye E, lens F, anterior focal length f.

Examples include: print enlargement, buying a large-screen television or using a large button telephone. Relative size magnification is further described in Chapter 10.

Angular magnification

Telescopes allow an image even in the far distance to be seen as larger by exploiting angular magnification. A sequence of lenses increases the angle of subtense of incoming light while the object distance remains constant.

Telescopes are described in detail in Chapter 8.

Electronic, digital or transverse magnification

This method of magnification is utilized in electronic vision enhancement systems (EVES), (previously known as CCTV systems), where an image is captured digitally and then reproduced upon a screen. EVES are described in more detail in Chapter 9.

Prescribing strategies

Whatever the method used to estimate the patient's task magnification, it is important to remember that it is simply a starting point and the amount of magnification that is actually prescribed will depend upon several other factors such as the location of scotomata, the presence of central distortion, etc.

After estimating the magnification required for the task, and making an assessment of visual performance, it is important to have a clear strategy for prescribing. Rumney differentiates patients into three distinct groups on the basis of their threshold visual performance: [23]

- Limited or no survival reading potential
- Survival reading potential but limited likelihood of fluency
- Clear survival reading potential with fluent reading possible if motivated

It is important to start with the survival reading first to assist independence. Following any success here, then fluent reading may be introduced later. More than one appointment may be necessary, with motivation being a strong indicator for success in those patients who have indicated a potentially good reading performance. Often a patient will return having tried the aid at home for a while and, pleased with its initial success with survival or spot reading, is motivated to take things onto another level.

The list below gives several factors that are relevant when considering the design of a device to demonstrate to the patient:

- Does the patient need a device that is hands free or spectacle mounted?
- Does the patient have the ability to hold their hand steady?
- Does the patient have ease of handling or is there any factor such as arthritis that will affect the ability to hold a hand-held device?
- Is there a need for a flat surface?
- Is a close working distance acceptable?
- Is there a need for portability?
- Is additional lighting necessary?
- Is cosmesis important to the patient?
- Will there be training involved?
- Is cost important?

Summary

It is important to remember that in the same way it is not always necessary to achieve 6/6, it is not always necessary to achieve N5. There is little point in giving the patient an excess of magnification to achieve N5 when N12 will do. Therefore, establishing a methodical approach to the assessment of tasks and magnification and taking into consideration the reserves of acuity and contrast etc. will result in a more realistic outcome for the patient.

It may not be possible to deal with all requests during the first visit, and similarly, it is often not possible to eliminate all fears or anxieties. A patient who initially appears satisfied and reassured after the first visit may not have revealed the whole picture. Ideally, allow the patient to try the aid at home for a while, and then bring them back to find out how they are managing, if the aid was indeed useful, and if any new problems are arising.

References

1. Massof RW, Ahmadian L, Grover LL, Deremeik JT, Goldstein JE, Rainey C, et al. The Activity Inventory: an adaptive visual function questionnaire. Optom Vis Sci. 2007;84(8):763–74.
2. Bruijning JE, van Rens GHMB, Knol DL, van Nispen RMA. evaluation of reading, writing, and watching TV using the Dutch ICF Activity Inventory. Optom Vis Sci. 2014;91(11):1360–71.
3. Latham K, Whitaker D. A comparison of word recognition and reading performace in foveal and peripheral vision. Vision Res. 1996;36(17):2665–74.
4. Lovie-Kitchin JE. Reading with low vision: The impact of research on clinical management. Clin Exp Optom. 2011;94(2):121–32.
5. Legge G, Mansfield J, Chung S. Psychophysics of reading. Clinical predictors of low-vision reading speed. Invest Ophthalmol Vis Sci. 1992;33:677–87.
6. Sloan L. New test charts for the measurement of visual acuity at far and near distances. Am J Ophthalmol. 1959;48:807–13.
7. Sloan L, Brown D. Reading cards for selection of optical aids for the partially sighted. Am J Ophthalmol. 1963;55(6):1187-1199.
8. Bailey IL, Lovie-Kitchin JE. The design and use of a new near vision chart. Am J Optom Physiol Opt. 1980;57(6):378–87.
9. Bailey IL. Optics of low vision magnifiers. Optom Pract. 2017;18(2):73–82.
10. Latham K, Tabrett DR. Guidelines for predicting performance with low vision aids. Optom Vis Sci. 2012;89(9):1316–26.
11. Ahn SJ, Legge G, Luebker A. Printed cards for measuring low-vision reading speed. Vision Res. 1995;35(13):1939–44.
12. Mansfield J, Legge G. The MNREAD acuity chart. Psychophysics of reading: normal low vision. 2007;167–91.
13. Legge G. MNREAD, Scoring for non-standard viewing distances [Internet]. 2011. Available from: http://legge.psych.umn.edu/mnread/acuity.html

14. Subramanian A, Pardhan S. The repeatability of MNREAD acuity charts and variability at different test distances. Optom Vis Sci. 2006;83(8):572–6.
15. Subramanian A, Pardhan S. Repeatability of reading ability indices in subjects with impaired vision. Investig Ophthalmol Vis Sci. 2009;50(8):3643–7.
16. Lovie-Kitchin JE, Brown B. Repeatability and intercorrelations of standard vision tests as a function of age. Optom Vis Sci. 2000;77(8):412–20.
17. Legge G, Pelli DG, Rubin GS, Schleske MM. Psychophysics of reading-I. Normal vision. Vision Res. 1985;25(2):239–52.
18. Whittaker SG, Lovie-Kitchin JE. Visual requirements for reading. Optom Vis Sci. 1993;70(1):54–65.
19. Lovie-Kitchin JE, Whittaker SG. Prescribing near magnification for low vision patients. Clin Exp Optom. 1999;82(6):214–24.
20. Legge G, Ross J, Luebker A, LaMay JM. Psychophysics of reading. VIII. The Minnesota Low-Vision Reading Test. Optom Vis Sci. 1989;66(12):843–53.
21. Mansfield J, Legge G. Psychophysics of reading XV: font effects in normal and low vision. Investig Ophthalmol Vis Sci. 1996;37(8):1492–501.
22. Whittaker S, Lovie-Kitchin J. The assessment of contrast sensitivity and contrast reserve for reading. Low Vis Res New Dev Rehabil. 1994;11(88).
23. Rumney N. Using visual thresholds to establish low vision performance. Ophthalmic Physiol Opt. 1995;C(1)18-24.

CHAPTER SIX

Hand & Stand Magnifiers

> “User acceptance of any low vision aid relies on many factors beyond its primary function. A patient-centred approach must be applied throughout the design process of any visual aid considering the target demographic and their challenges.”

Stuart Baldwin, Director Associated Optical

Hand & Stand Magnifiers

The importance of good design

There is a wealth of products on the market that claim to assist people with a visual impairment. But choosing a long-term, successful product for a patient is not always straightforward and requires a review of the patient's clinical, refractive and psychological status. Using a magnification device is almost always a compromise compared to 'standard' reading glasses, yet it is a compromise many patients are willing to make especially when it can return a degree of previously lost independence. However, all too often motivated patients are let down by a poorly designed or poorly manufactured product. The objective of this chapter is to outline the generic design features of hand and stand magnifiers and to highlight what makes a low vision aid successful and ultimately an indispensable lifeline to a patient.

In recent years, there have been a number of exciting new products entering the marketplace. Successful manufacturers have invested wisely in not just good product components and design but have held discussions with focus groups and end-users who review the functionality of the product. If a patient with low vision uses additional magnification to do basic daily tasks, then arguably they should expect their magnifier to have the same quality optics as a spectacle lens. There are cheaper products that appear within the marketplace, offering inferior quality lenses with distortion or aberrations and casing that becomes brittle or discoloured over a short time period. Similarly, there are products boasting a high-quality lens with a superb ergonomic handle but other features such as a fiddly battery compartment or a flimsy switch mechanism let the product down. As a prescriber, it is useful to have time to review the products carefully and be reminded that what may appear useful for a sighted individual may not be as useful for someone suffering from a visual impairment.

Lens power and lens form

With such a wide variety of hand and stand magnifiers available in the marketplace containing spherical, biconvex, aspheric or aplanatic lenses, it is important that practitioners take time to consider the benefits of each with their visually impaired users or hobbyists in mind.

Single lens powers for optical devices range from approximately +4.00D to over +50D and lens quality can vary significantly between product ranges. Most devices contain just the one lens although some hand or stand magnifiers may contain a double lens system to either increase overall magnification, field of view, or both. At the lower powers, magnifiers can afford to have a larger lens diameter. Standard spherical lenses tend to be used in the economy ranges but will suffer from aberration and distortion in the higher powers. Biconvex lenses offer larger lens diameters, particularly in the lower power range and if the patient requires stronger magnification, using an aspheric lens will go some way to reduce weight and thickness whilst controlling distortion and aberrations such as oblique astigmatism.

As mentioned in Chapter 5, a significant factor influencing reading performance is the field of view through the lens.[1] In the higher powers (>24D approx.), the overall diameter of the lens is significantly reduced and therefore practitioners need to assist patients in realising their personal expectations with reading fluency when using a device with a restricted field of view.

Within the marketplace, an aplanatic lens may offer a slightly wider field of view. An aplanatic 'lens' consists of two lenses, such as a plano-convex bonded together to produce a doublet to reduce spherical aberration and coma.

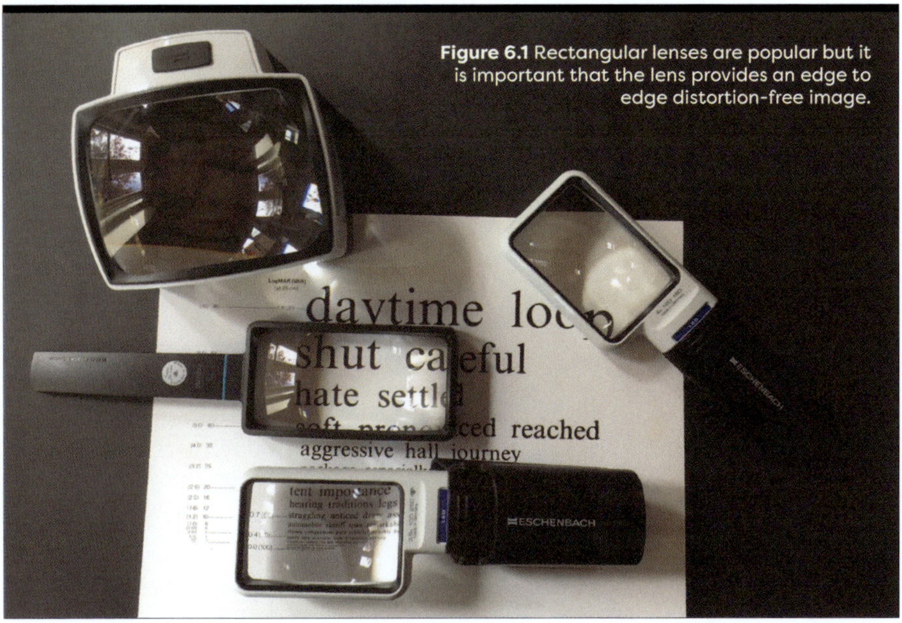

Figure 6.1 Rectangular lenses are popular but it is important that the lens provides an edge to edge distortion-free image.

In the lower power range, there is also the option to create a larger, rectangular lens, and maintain good quality optics. A rectangular lens is useful for those who are reading a line or a column of newspaper print, (Figure 6.1). Several factors, including weight, lens quality and cost restrict the manufacture of a usable aspheric rectangular lens beyond approximately +10D as a low vision device, unless the lens is created by multi-order diffractive (MOD) optics, (Figure 6.2).

One or two manufacturers have produced rectangular lens claiming a wider field of view by creating a form of 'blended' lens, where the stated power is only central to the lens (often termed the 'usable area') and the lens power tapers off towards the lens edge. This lens design may not be beneficial for patients with central vision loss or central distortion, who require an edge-to-edge distortion free lens as they move their eyes around to capture an eccentric view of the text or image.

Multi-order diffractive aspheric lenses (MOD) have been introduced in several low vision devices, offering

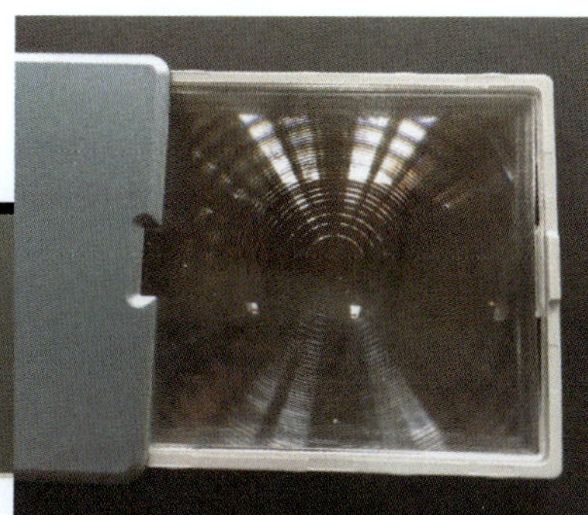

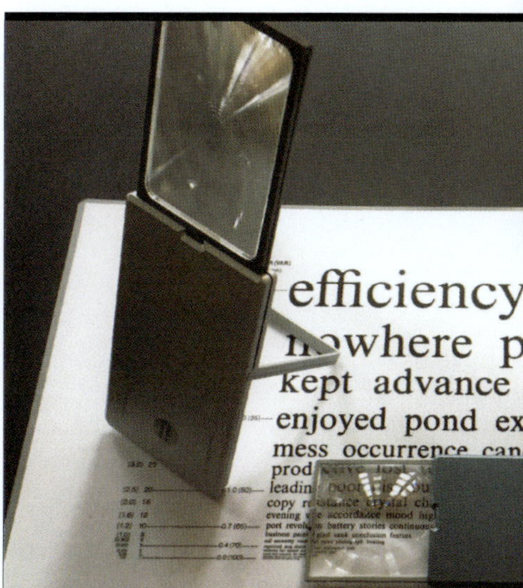
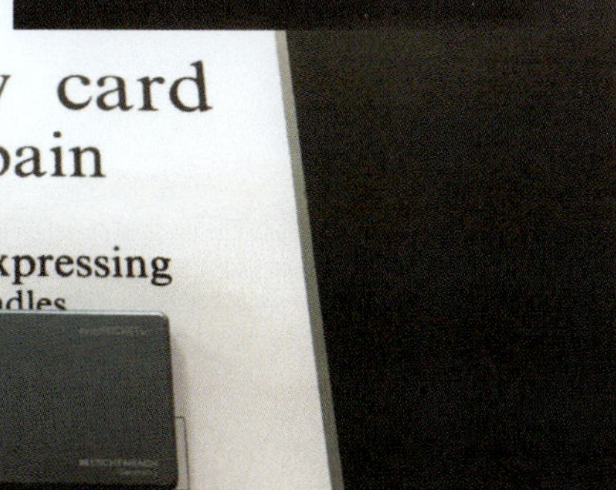

Figure 6.2 *Eschenbach's* Easy Pocket. Illuminated ultra thin magnifiers produced by multi-order diffractive optics.

higher-powered lenses for both hand-held devices and high-powered spectacles with a significant reduction in weight and thickness compared to similar powered aspheric lens designs. They also boast excellent quality optics but should not be mistaken for the familiar Fresnel lenses used in low-cost 'sheet' magnifiers, which offer limited magnification and which come with poor quality optics and significant chromatic aberration.

Adding to the lens quality, it is also practical to have a lens that is hard coated. Devices are carried about loosely in bags and pockets, rather than within boxes or in pouches for quick, easy access at all times. Devices using lenses that scratch easily do not last long. Those with a visual impairment may not be aware of lens degradation and may wrongly assume they have experienced a drop in vision. In those lens designs that are unable to have a hard coating, practitioners need to inform users that additional care may be taken when handling or transporting the device.

Handle ergonomics

With older users in mind, handle shape and thickness is an important feature for those with weak or arthritic hands. An ergonomic handle with a simple or smooth switch mechanism is preferable in a material that is easy to wipe clean and ideally with contrasting colours that improve the device's visibility around the home. Some manufacturers use antibacterial plastics materials and one or two have produced a hand magnifier with 'auto-touch' mechanisms where the magnifier illuminates only when held in the hand.

LED Illumination

By far the vast majority of illuminated devices used in low vision benefit from an LED (light emitting diode) light source. LED's emit more light per watt than previously used incandescent light bulbs (Tungsten/Tungsten-Halogen) and are more energy efficient, radiating very little heat. Furthermore, efficiency is not affected by shape or size so LED's can be incorporated easily within a device without adding extra weight or bulk. An LED will light up very quickly, achieving full brightness in under a microsecond and has estimated between 35,000 to 50,000 hours of useful life. Before LED's became the norm, previously used incandescent bulbs had between 1,000–2,000 hours of useful life and were less energy efficient, radiating a noticeable amount of heat.

Being made of solid-state components, LED's are less susceptible to external shock, unlike the more fragile incandescent bulbs, useful when the devices are carried in bags and pockets.

Some product ranges now incorporate a surface-mounted, (SMD) LED consisting of an LED that is soldered directly onto a circuit board (Figure 6.3) With no leads or surrounding 'packaging' that comes with a standard LED, weight and bulk are further reduced. The SMD LED gives off almost no heat and has very low voltage and low current requirements. SMD LED's have an extended life span estimated at 100,000 hrs. Some products that incorporate SMD LED's will additionally use a step-up converter to ensure consistent illumination over time so when the voltage drops near the end of battery life, the light dims quickly, and may even flicker, giving the user clear indication when to replace the batteries.

Integral illumination is an essential feature for many users with low vision; attention should therefore be given to the position of the LED within the design. To maximise field of view, many users hold their device close to the eye, therefore it is important to have the light source concealed from view to avoid causing a glare source whilst at the same time also ensuring that the position of the LED is not in a location where it is covered by hands or fingers when in use. An ideal light source should create even illumination across the entire field of view. To achieve this, one or two product lines house the LED within a collimator (Figure 6.3).

There have been few studies that have looked into the benefits of different correlated color temperatures (CCT) in low vision devices and there is no current evidence to suggest that there is an improved reading performance using one specific colour temperature over another.[2] Anecdotally however, low vision practitioners are aware there are undoubtedly subjective preferences between users, therefore it is important to consider demonstrating all colour temperature options where possible. Manufacturers offer alternative colour temperatures from approximately 2,500K (warm white) to 8,000K (cold white) or higher in their more popular ranges of hand or stand devices. Products offering a range of colour temperatures are available as either separate devices or one single device offering filters that are simply clipped over the LED (Figure 6.3).

Batteries and battery compartments

Although the use of an LED/SMD LED adds little weight, the batteries most certainly do. Smaller batteries are often more difficult for older patients to hold and change and ideally, they should be readily available as many older or infirm patients are less likely to travel far or shop on the internet for less commonly used replacements. The battery compartment should be simple to open and close and be robust enough to withstand heavy handling. Insertion and removal of batteries should be intuitive as many patients may not be able to see well enough and will 'feel' their way around when trying to open the casing, assuming that the contact springs will indicate battery direction. All too often a design is let down by ignoring these important features when marketing a device to a person with visual impairment. If a patient is unable to change the batteries, the device will end up unused and in a kitchen drawer.

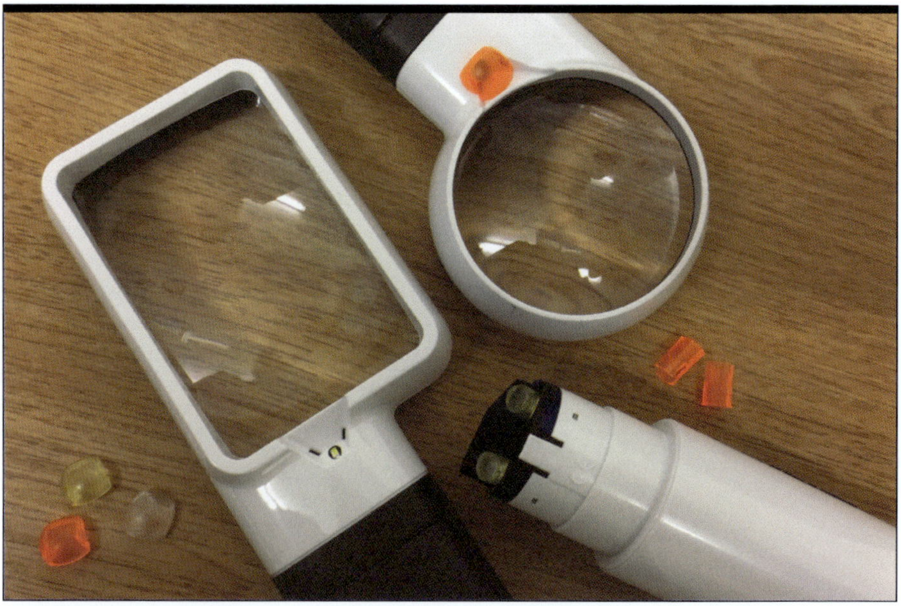

Figure 6.3 Interchangeable clip on collimators attach over the surface-mounted LED of these hand magnifiers to provide even illumination with a range of CCT (6500K to 3400K). Interchangeable filters for the stand magnifier handle (bottom right) provide a CCT range from 8000K to 3400K.

With a good quality lens, several designs are let down by poor quality casing. Ideally, the aid should have a durable casing that adds little weight. Several products in the marketplace are prone to discolouration, especially if the patient is a smoker. Others become brittle and crack over a relatively short time.

Choosing the best device

Once the task and level of magnification has been established, the next step is to demonstrate aids of appropriate type and design to meet the patient's needs. For example, if the patient needs something to help see the prices of goods in a supermarket, then a hand-held portable device is a good option with which to start. It is also preferable to narrow the initial choice of aids to a few, and thus avoid the frustration of going through a number of unsuitable devices, which may be upsetting for the patient.

The aim is to prescribe the minimum magnification with the maximum acceptable field of view wherever possible, taking into consideration the need for any acuity reserve as discussed in Chapter 5. Both field of view and working distance are rapidly compromised at higher levels of magnification, therefore it follows that prescribing excess magnification will be unconstructive. For example, the magnification required to read a large print book compared to a newspaper will be different. If the patient regularly carries out both tasks, then perhaps two magnifiers of different strengths would be sensible.

The response to a low vision device will emerge quickly during the consultation. Using an aid may be a constant reminder that the vision is not as good as what it used to be. The psychological impact of vision loss is covered in more detail in Chapter 12 and has a significant influence on the initial response to using a device. For example, those who have a greater acceptance of their vision loss are more likely to be motivated to try something new. Other factors such as cognitive or physical impairments will also influence the initial choice of aid.

Hand magnifiers

Within any low vision service, hand magnifiers continue to be the most popular choice of aid, being readily available and familiar.[3] They are portable and are more acceptable cosmetically to many older patients. Many feel that using a hand magnifier in public is less likely to draw attention compared with using a spectacle-mounted telescope. Whether bought in a junk shop or found in amongst the old stamp collection, almost all patients who have suffered a visual impairment will have tried using one in one form or another and long before any formal low vision assessment. It is often useful to ask the patient to bring their old hand magnifier with them to an assessment, even if they are finding it difficult to use. Comparisons with better equipment can be swiftly made. In addition, it is not unusual to simply increase the reading addition in their current spectacles so that the same magnifiers may be used with greater efficiency (see: equivalent power, below).

Although one hand is used up during use, hand magnifiers offer the most flexibility, both within the home and out and about and *either* pair of spectacles may be worn, distance *or* near (see below). Hand magnifiers are easier to use when the task is in a less accessible place or position, such as such as a washing machine dial particularly when the patient has a variable head position and working distance; hand magnifiers are also easier to use when viewing text on a curved or variable surface such as viewing ingredients on food tins or packets.

Stand magnifiers

In using a stand magnifier, the fixed lens-object working distance gives a more stable image, useful for those who struggle to keep a steady hand. Due to the fixed working distance, text is kept in focus and the patient can leave the device over the object and come back to it later. As a result, patients may be able to use higher ranges of magnification with greater ease than with the similar powered hand magnifier. Popular designs include handled stand magnifiers, which have a good sturdy handle housing the batteries (Figure 6.4). Weight becomes less of an issue as the device is placed directly over the object. Visual tracking is aided in some designs with the incorporation of an additional reading line, which can be moved out of view when not required.

Larger diameter lenses that have a longer focal length may be used for writing (Figure 6.5) and some designs are shaped to assist a comfortable hand position (Figure 6.6). Double lens systems also have the benefits of increasing magnification and maintaining a larger field of view (Figure 6.6). These lens systems are not to be confused with telescopes in which lenses are separated by a defined distance based upon their focal lengths.

One major disadvantage of using either a hand magnifier or a stand magnifier is that one hand is used in the process. The aid has to travel across the page and so the text is usually put on a flat surface such as a table or a clipboard. A sturdy reading stand with a variety of tilting positions, offers an improvement on reading posture, and may also be useful for those struggling to achieve the shorter eye-lens working distance of a higher-powered device (Figure 6.7).

Using magnification for substantial volumes of text is often tiring or frustrating. When using the higher-powered magnifiers, the field of view will be quite restrictive and patients often complain of only being able to read one word at a time and may lose the context or meaning of the passage.

From a practical viewpoint, hand and stand magnifiers are popular due to their familiarity and ease of use. For those who suffer from dementia, familiarity is an important consideration when prescribing. Learning a new technique may not be realistic, therefore having a device that uses a skill previously learned is of particular importance.

Spectacle correction

If the lens-object distance is set within the focal length of the lens or lens system, then the emergent vergence entering the patient's eye will be slightly divergent. This means that the patient will need to either accommodate to focus the image on the retina or use a spectacle reading addition. If the lens is placed at its focal length from the object then the emergent vergence of the overall system is now 0 dioptres and parallel; the patient will not require additional accommodation or a reading addition and will need to wear a distance correction, if they have one.

The use of a hand magnifier is a dynamic system. The patient will alter the position of the magnifier lens from the object to create the correct level of vergence needed according to which pair of spectacles they have chosen to wear. When wearing a distance correction, the patient will adjust the position of the lens closer to its focal length; when wearing a reading correction, the patient will adjust the position of the lens closer to the object.

When using a stand magnifier, the emergent vergence of the overall system is fixed. When a stand magnifier design has a lens set close to its focal length,

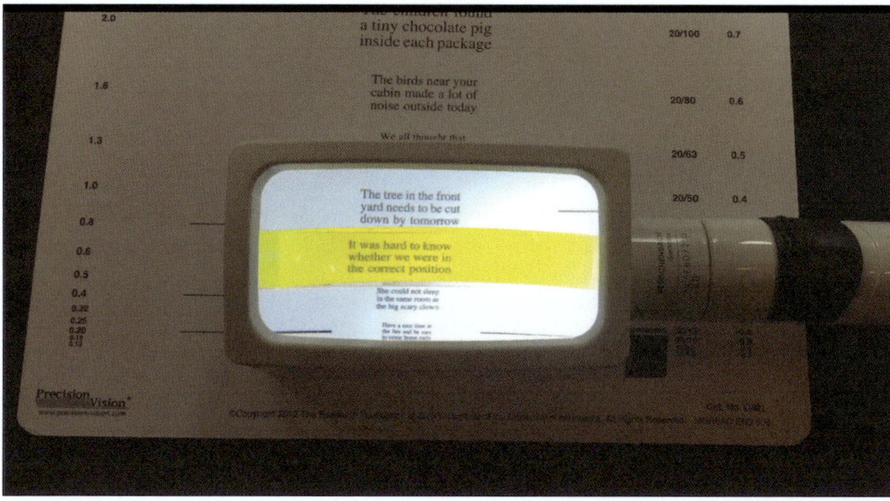

Figure 6.4 +7.6D Handled stand magnifier with tilted head and an additional +4D high contrast retractable lens.

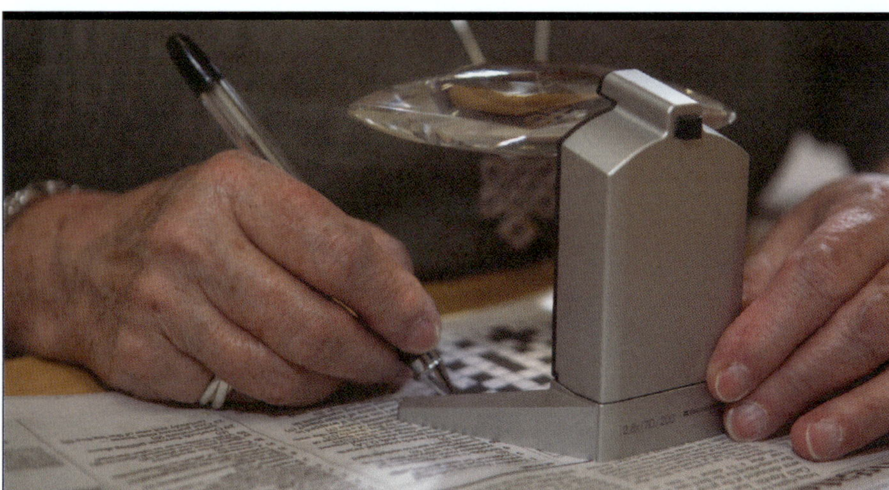

Figure 6.5 An illuminated stand magnifier being used with a pen – useful for form-filling or puzzles.

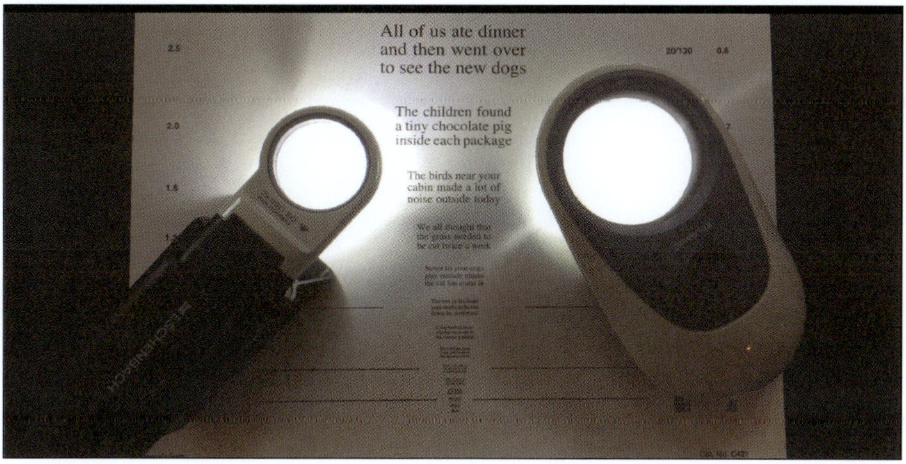

Figure 6.6 An ergonomic stand magnifier based upon the shape of a familiar computer mouse (*right*). A double lens system creates 7x magnification (+28D) with an overall diameter of 58mm. The equivalent single lens 7x (+28D) hand magnifier (*left*) has a diameter of 35mm.

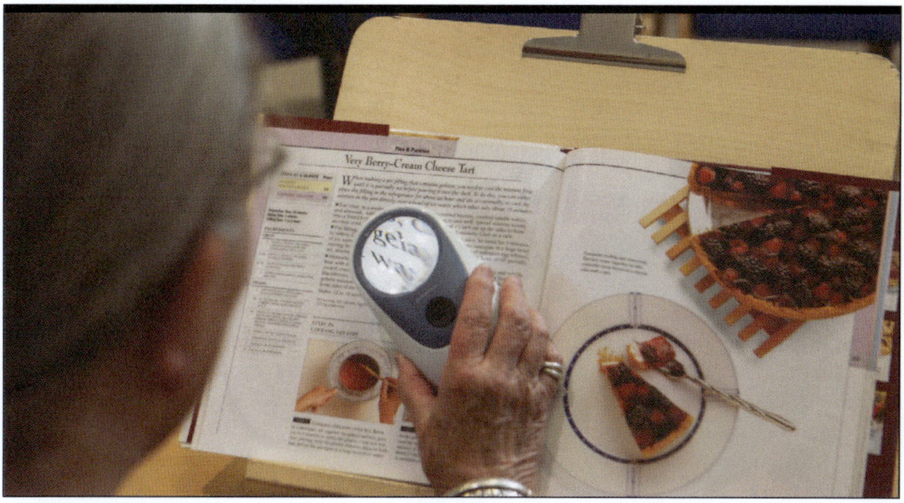

Figure 6.7 The use of a reading stand can create a more comfortable reading posture.

the emergent vergence entering the eye will be close to 0 dioptres. Therefore, a distance correction will be more suitable.

However, many stand magnifier designs have the lens-object distance set within its focal length, so that a reading addition (or accommodative effort) is needed to correct for the vergence of the light entering the eye. How much vergence varies between manufacturers and with the power of the lens, and may range, for example, between 1.50D to 3.00D. Practitioners need to be aware of the differences so that they may advise their patients on the best spectacle correction to use in conjunction with the device. Practitioners are therefore directed to the manufacturer on which reading addition is recommended. It is therefore important to remind patients to keep hold of their old reading glasses for use with these devices.

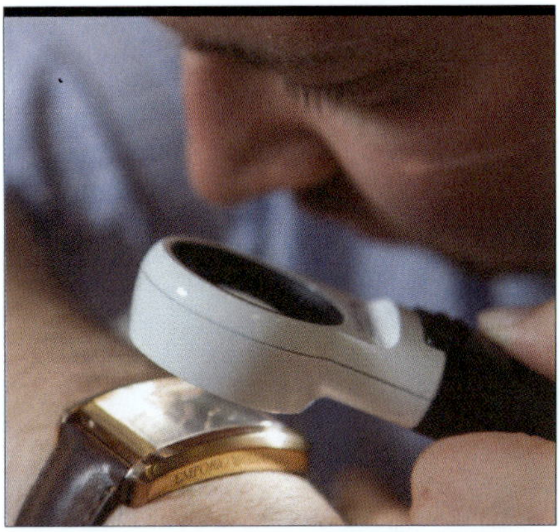

Fig 6.8 To improve the field of view the user is encouraged to reduce the eye-lens working distance.

Field of view and equivalent power

Most patients benefit from the additional practical advice from practitioners to get the most out of the aid in particular improving both the field of view and equivalent power by reducing the lens-eye working distance (Figure 6.8). The magnifier should be moved away from the object viewed until a clear image is found. Keeping this aid-to-object distance constant, the eye may then be moved closer to the magnifier to improve the field of view. This also has a bearing on the magnification achieved. When using a reading correction, the reading addition in the spectacles will also impact upon overall magnification. The equivalent power of the system, Fe, is equal to the sum of the powers of the reading add (Fa) and the magnifier (Fm) minus the product of the two powers and the separation between them (z), thus:

Equivalent power

$$Fe = Fa + Fm - (zFaFm)$$

Example: In Figure 6.9, the spectacle lens reading addition is +2.50D and the magnifier power is +10.00D. In Figure 6.9a, the separation between the spectacle addition and the magnifier lens is 5cm (z=0.05m). The equivalent power will therefore be:

$$Fa + Fm - (zFaFm) = 2.50 + 10 - (0.05 \times 2.50 \times 10) = 11.25D$$

If z is zero (Figure 6.9b) then the equivalent power will be +12.50D. Only when z gets larger does the magnification reduce. Therefore, the maximum magnification and field of view is gained when the lens is held up against the spectacle addition. In the higher powers, this distance becomes more critical. If the patient in Figure 6.9 were to use a +38D magnifier, the equivalent power held at 5cm would be +35.75D, compared with +40.50D at 0cm. Therefore, equivalent power and thus the magnification achieved from using a device will vary depending upon how it is used rather than what is printed on the side of the box it originally came in. Encourage patients to improve both field of view and level of magnification achieved from the device by adopting a short working distance.

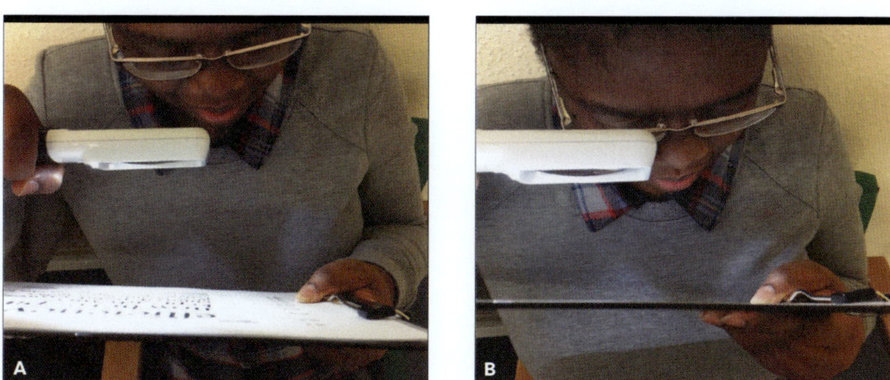

Fig 6.9 The patient's spectacle reading addition is +2.50D and the magni er power is +10.00D. **A)** less magnification is achieved when the separation between the spectacle lens and the magnifier increases **B)** Maximum field of view and magnification are achieved when the spectacle lens and magnifier have a separation of 0.

Adapting hand-held to hands-free

The term 'hands-free' means different things to different people. For some, the term 'hands-free' means having the full use of both hands to hold a book or a paper, rather than holding a device and moving it across the page. Such adaptations either offer the full use of both hands to perform a specific task, or to allow the user to adopt a more natural reading posture.

Stands and Clamps

There are a few products that have created either an integrated or a removable stand for a hand magnifier so converting to a stand magnifier when needed. This offers even more flexibility of use with little additional cost. For example, the hand magnifier may incorporate foldaway metal legs that can be used to create a tilted stand for a comfortable viewing experience; alternative designs offer an additional stand attachment into which the hand magnifier may be placed or inserted (Figures 6.10 and 6.11).

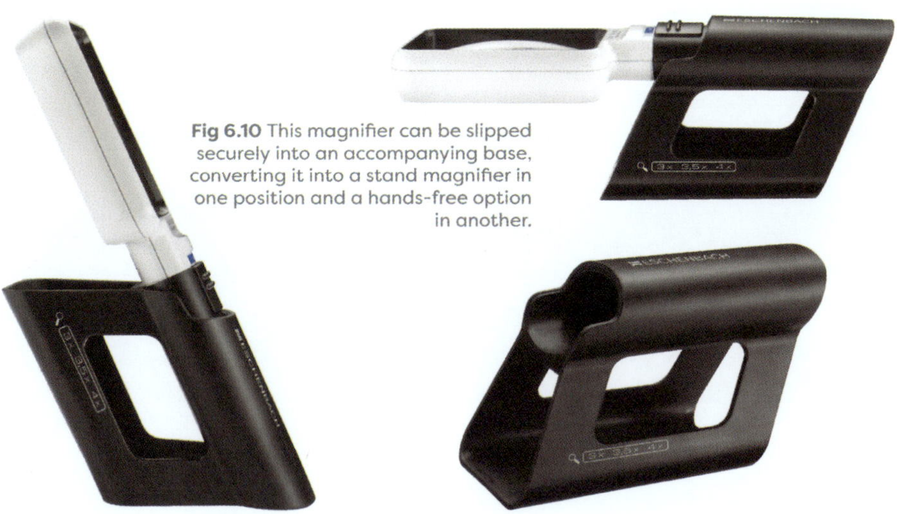

Fig 6.10 This magnifier can be slipped securely into an accompanying base, converting it into a stand magnifier in one position and a hands-free option in another.

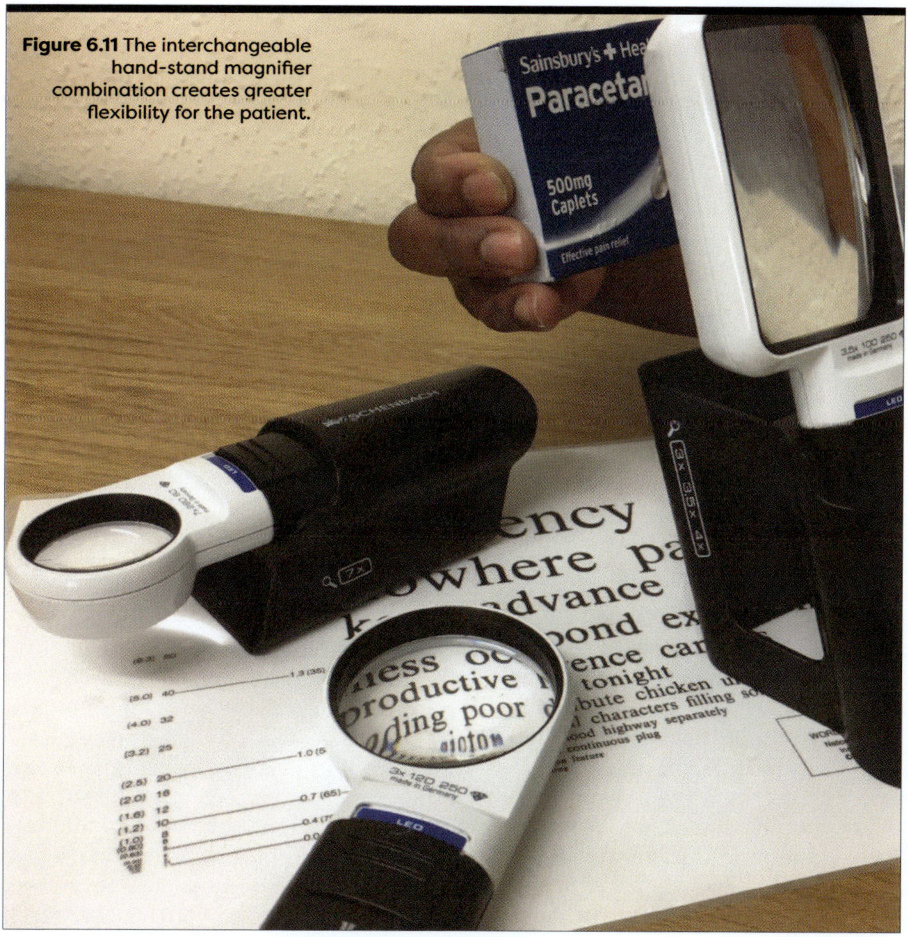

Figure 6.11 The interchangeable hand-stand magnifier combination creates greater flexibility for the patient.

One of the simplest methods to create a hands-free solution is to clamp a standard magnifier into a flexible or adjustable stand so that the hands may hold the object beneath it (Figure 6.12). Most handled magnifiers can be securely slipped into a sturdy double-ended clamp and moved into position for the task. When choosing a stand for this purpose, the clamps at either must be strong and the stand is both flexible enough to place into position but sturdy enough the take the weight of the device.

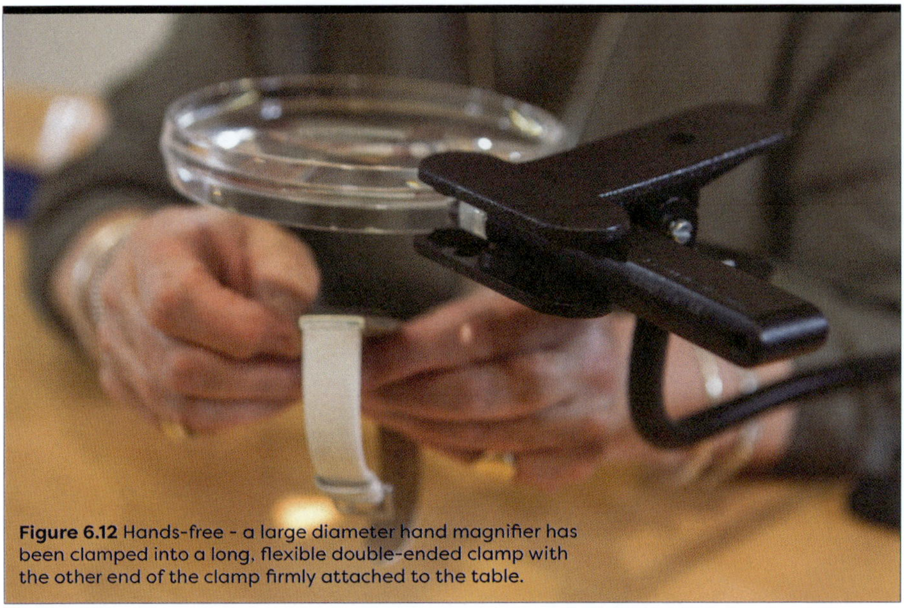

Figure 6.12 Hands-free - a large diameter hand magnifier has been clamped into a long, flexible double-ended clamp with the other end of the clamp firmly attached to the table.

Desk-top illuminated table clamp magnifiers offer the same flexibility as a double-ended clamp but with the advantage of additional lighting (Figure 6.13). Offering low to medium levels of magnification and with a long flexible stand, these relatively large diameter lenses may either be clamped securely onto the desk or table or come as free-standing units with a heavy base to offer stability. The user may wear either their distance or near spectacle correction and the object is moved into the right point beneath the magnifier. Suspended magnifiers (also termed neck or chest magnifiers) are typically low powered and lightweight and are suspended around the patient's neck by a simple cord, with feet resting on the patient's chest (Figure 6.14). These types of magnifier are used by both people with a visual impairment and hobbyists who seek a hands-free solution for common tasks such as knitting or crafts. As the lens diameter is quite large, lens powers tend to be low although many lens designs will have a higher-powered 'insert' of a small diameter to assist with detail when required. Similar to the flexible clamp solution, the patient may wear either their distance or near spectacle correction and then adjust the position of the hands beneath the magnifier to find the appropriate focusing distance.

Figure 6.13 Table clamp magnifiers such as this one offer hands-free magnification thanks to the long, flexible stand length. This model offers 2.5x magnification with the advantage of additional LED task lighting.

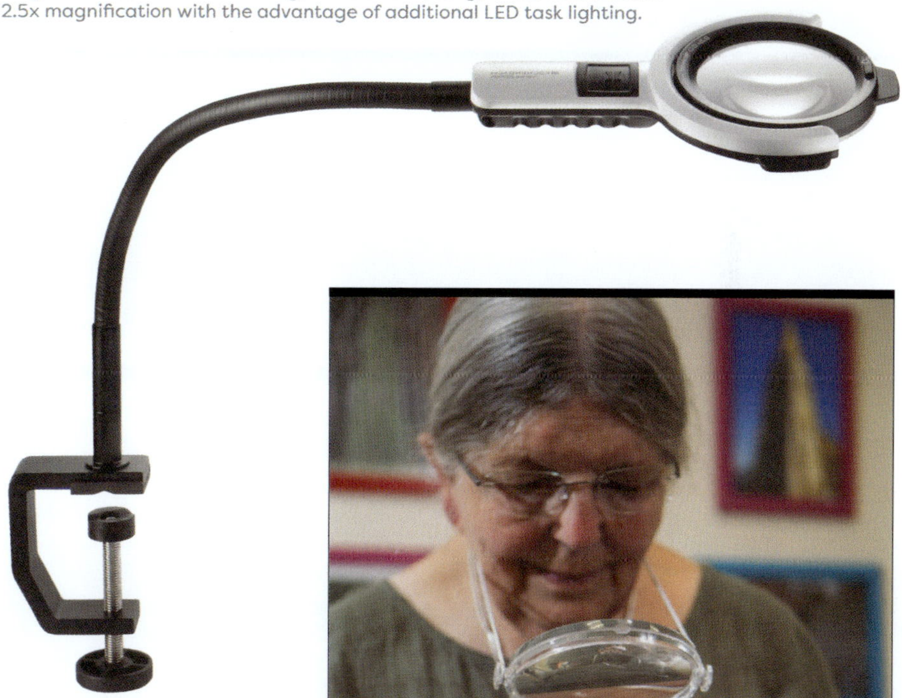

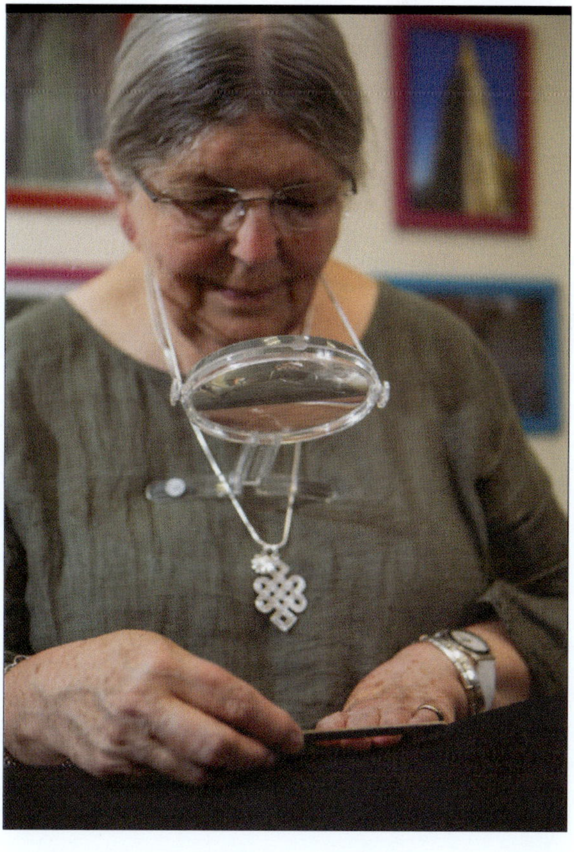

Figure 6.14 The patient is using a 2x suspended magnifier. The feet have rubberised or foam pads that stop the magnifier from slipping over the user's clothing and thetransparent frame reduces unwanted shadows allowing for more light to reach the task.

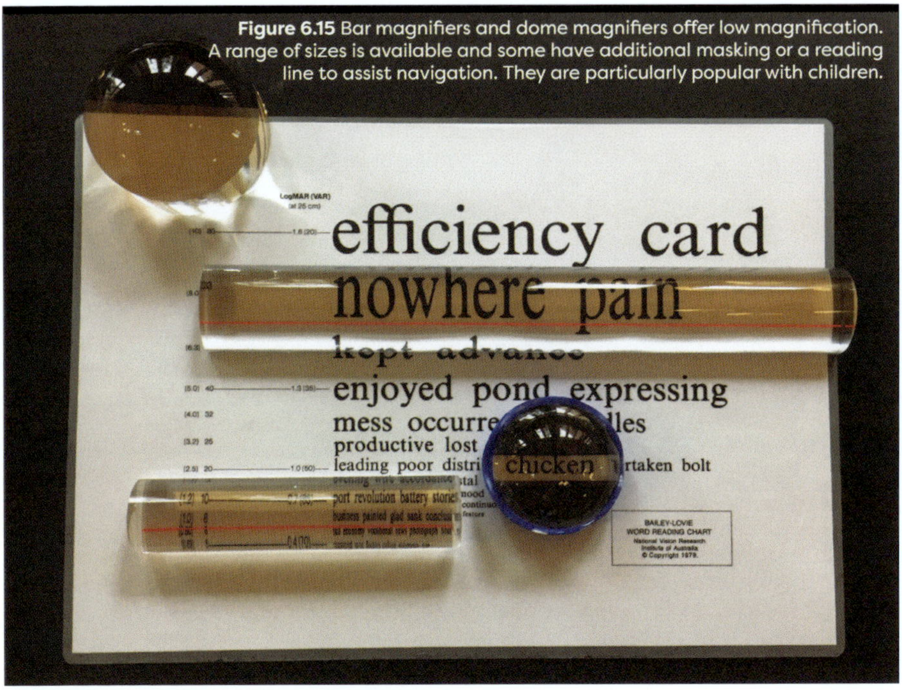

Figure 6.15 Bar magnifiers and dome magnifiers offer low magnification. A range of sizes is available and some have additional masking or a reading line to assist navigation. They are particularly popular with children.

Bright-field magnifiers

The term 'bright-field' (also known as flat-field) refers to a range of aids where the lens is placed directly onto the reading material or object in view and the image created has the same field of view regardless of the eye-lens working distance. Therefore, there is negligible change in the field of view by moving in closer to the lens compared to using a hand or stand magnifier. These devices offer the user an improvement in posture when in use and a binocular view. Although this type of aid is only available in the lower powers, several designs are available from the popular 'dome' magnifiers, (Figure 6.15) to those that have successfully incorporated additional illumination (Figure 6.16). The magnification produced by this type of device is usually 1.5x-2x although some designs have used additional lenses or have encased the lens slightly off the page to create additional magnification.

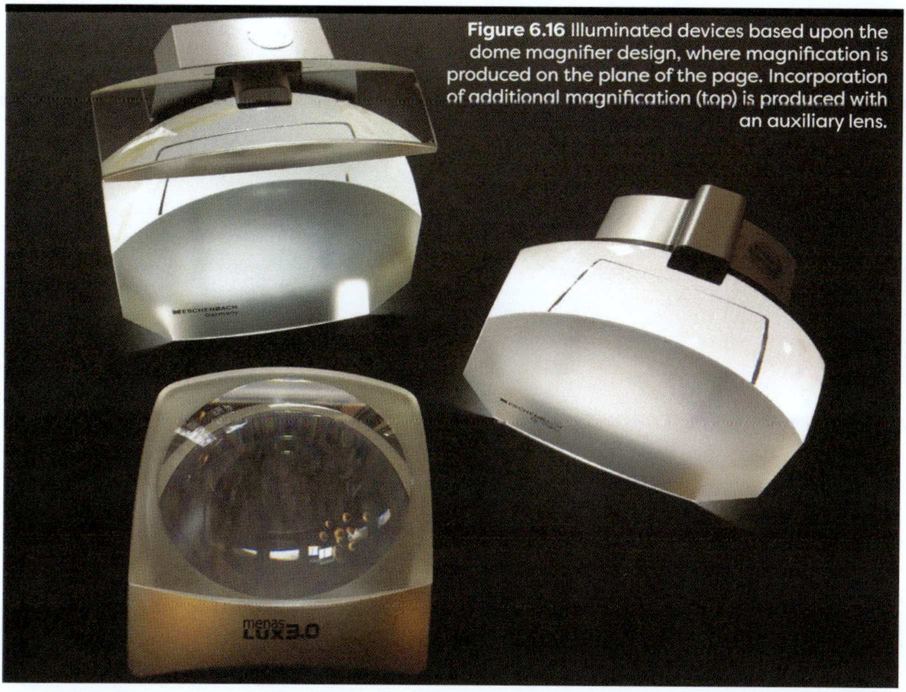

Figure 6.16 Illuminated devices based upon the dome magnifier design, where magnification is produced on the plane of the page. Incorporation of additional magnification (top) is produced with an auxiliary lens.

As the magnification produced is on the plane of the page, a reading addition or accommodative effort for the working distance at which the page is held will produce the clearest image for the user. Reducing the eye-lens viewing distance further, the patient will benefit from the additional relative distance magnification that this creates, which is one of the reason why this type of device works well with children who have good levels of accommodation. In recent years, these devices have become more popular as lightweight acrylic materials have produced robust and relatively inexpensive devices.[3]

Although 'bar' magnifiers offer the patient magnification across the whole line of a page, the magnification is produced in the vertical meridian only through the use of a sphero-cylindrical lens. This type of device tends to be less popular when used by both adults or children with low vision, who prefer an undistorted magnified image of the text or object.

Summary

Although some health and social care services are still concerned that optical magnifiers can be expensive, the additional enhancement on vision may be priceless for the patient. Using a device of any nature is always a compromise to the previous experience of being able to read a book on a lap, yet for many patients a simple magnifier can be a lifeline. The use of a device is a cost effective intervention and an important part of a multidisciplinary rehabilitation process; low vision devices greatly reduce both the social and economic impact of low vision.[4,5]

References

1. Whittaker SG, Lovie-Kitchin JE. Visual requirements for reading. Optom Vis Sci. 1993;70(1):54–65.
2. Wolffsohn JS, Palmer E, Rubinstein M, Eperjesi F. Effect of light-emitting diode colour temperature on magnifier reading performance of the visually impaired. Clin Exp Optom. 2012;95(5):510–4.
3. Crossland MD, Silver JH. Thirty years in an urban low vision clinic: changes in prescribing habits of low vision practitioners. Optom Vis Sci. 2005;82(7):617–22.
4. Margrain TH. Minimising the impact of visual impairment: low vision aids are a simple way of alleviating impairment. Br Med J. 1999;318:1504.
5. Rabiee P, Parker G, Bernard S, Baxter K. Vision rehabilitation services: What is the evidence? University of York; 2015. p. 1-301.

The author would like to thank *Associated Optical* for the equipment and images within this chapter.

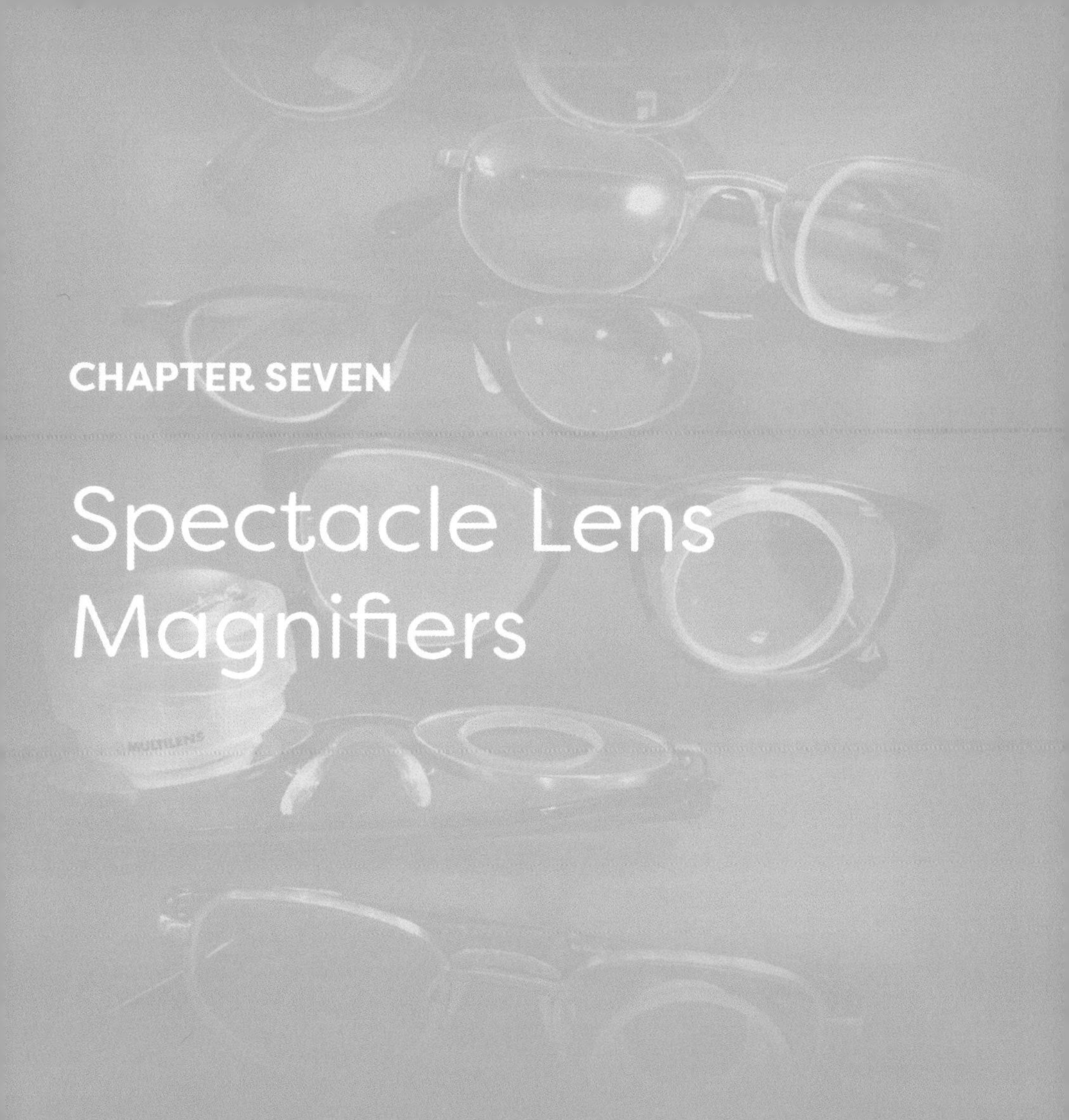

CHAPTER SEVEN

Spectacle Lens Magnifiers

> "Spectacle mounted aids are invaluable to our patients. The ability to have both hands free allows more freedom to achieve more tasks, returning a degree of independence and improving the scope for normal lives. They should not be forgotten by the practitioner."
>
> **Helen Denton FBDO (Hons) LVA Prof Cert LV**

Spectacle Lens Magnifiers

'Hands-free'

Many patients seek a 'hands-free' option rather than having to hold a device and move it across the page. Patients with arthritis in the neck or fingers, for example, or with muscle weakness affecting manual dexterity may opt to use hand-held devices for more essential spot-tasks such as cooking instructions on food packets or checking the dials of a cooker, where use tends to be relatively brief and thus less tiring. For sustained viewing tasks, such as reading a newspaper or sewing, spectacle mounted devices, offer a 'hands-free' option.

Definition

There are two main methods of incorporating spectacle-based magnification:

- Spectacle (lens) magnifiers and
- Spectacle-mounted or spectacle-based telescopes.

The term 'spectacle magnifier' often has a number of different definitions across manufacturers. For the purpose of this text however, spectacle magnification will refer directly to the addition or incorporation of plus lens power in the spectacle plane, producing relative distance magnification as discussed in Chapter 5. The patient will therefore be working at or slightly within the focal length of the plus lens. For example, in Figure 7.4 (see later) an emmetropic patient is wearing a 3x (+12D) spectacle magnifier. The distance at which she will need to hold the object or text is approximately 8.3cm from the spectacle plane.

Low vision practitioners are used to hearing requests from new patients on the possibility of 'stronger glasses.' The challenge the practitioner faces is to successfully demonstrate and convince the patient that the more powerful the plus lens in the spectacle plane, the shorter the working distance will be.

Devices that some manufacturers label as spectacle magnifiers, such as the popular TV Magnifiers seen in Figure 8.12 are more accurately classified as a telescope and are therefore discussed within Chapter 8. These devices utilise telescopic or angular magnification to extend the patient's working distance *beyond* the focal length of the equivalent powered spectacle lens magnifier thus offering the patient an extended working distance.

Monocular spectacle magnifiers

The additional plus power of a spectacle magnifier may be incorporated into the patient's distance prescription and ordered as a standard single vision or lenticulated higher plus lens from a prescription house in the usual way and may be glazed as a full or half eye to suit the patient.

High-plus lens forms

There is a modest number of spectacle lens forms available from various prescription houses and low vision suppliers including patented and trademarked lenses offering low to high levels of magnification. Some may also incorporate cylindrical correction. For an up-to-date range of availability, the practitioner should contact the suppliers for information.

Hyperocular lenses

Hyperocular lenses are lenticulated, biconvex aspheric lenses available from several prescription houses (Figures 7.1 and 7.2). They can be ordered as 'ready-made' spectacles glazed in a full-eye or half-eye format or are available as uncuts. They are injection moulded PMMA lenses and as such may not be tinted or coated. In ready-made formats the fellow eye may be glazed with a plano or occlusive lens to assist binocular comfort.

Segments and buttons

Single lenses and buttons may be added onto the patient's habitual correction or into a carrier mounting using a number of methods. For example, preformed lens segments may be screwed into a carrier that is either cemented onto the front surface of the patient's spectacles or into a separate self-adhesive mount. Interchangeable systems such as these are useful if the patient's vision is variable and when mounted onto the front surface of the patient's habitual correction, will allow for a cylinder to be corrected. If the habitual correction is not required then the segment may be screwed directly into an aperture cut out of a plano carrier that has been glazed within the spectacle frame. The interchangeable nature of such solutions offers flexibility in power change, are simple to put together, and reduce chair time and overall costs to both practitioner and patient.

An example of a more permanent solution is shown in Figure 7.3. The addition of a small plus-powered button is added directly onto the patient's habitual correction.

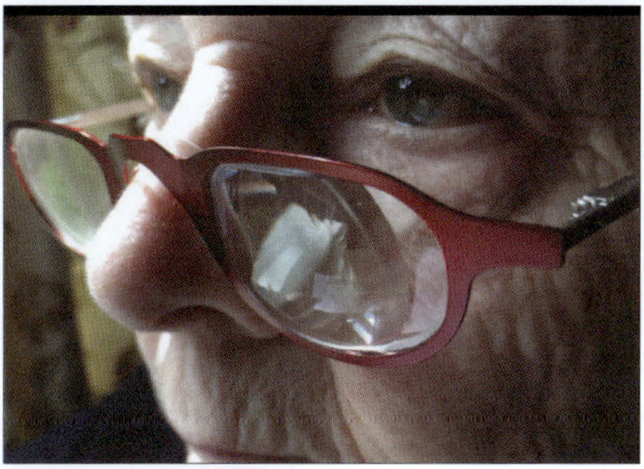

Figure 7.1 The patient is wearing a +16D hyperocular lens in the L eye from *Multilens.* The fellow eye has been lightly frosted to assist binocular comfort. The lenses have been glazed in a lightweight half-eye frame.

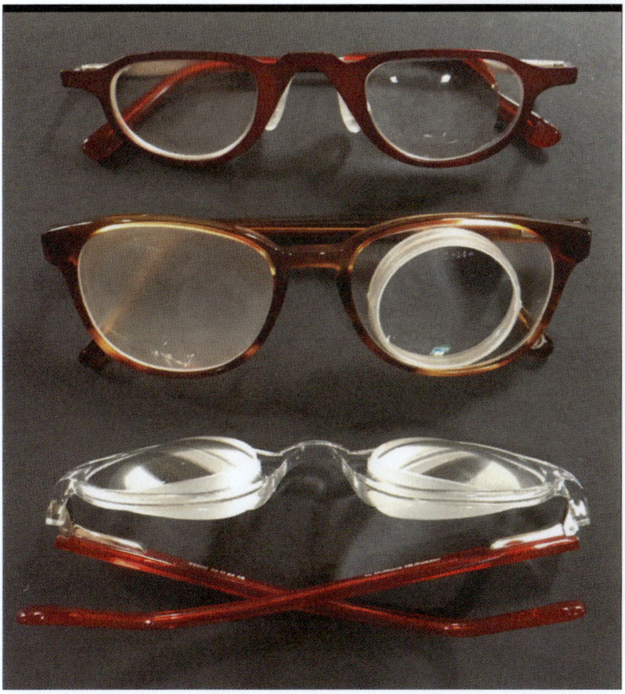

Figure 7.2 Three spectacle lens magnifiers from *Multilens*
Top: a 5x (+20D) hyperocular lens is set in the left eye in a half eye frame.
Middle: A flexible system consisting of an interchangeable aplanatic doublet that creates high levels of magnification without compromising the field of view.
Bottom: Half eye prismatic spectacles

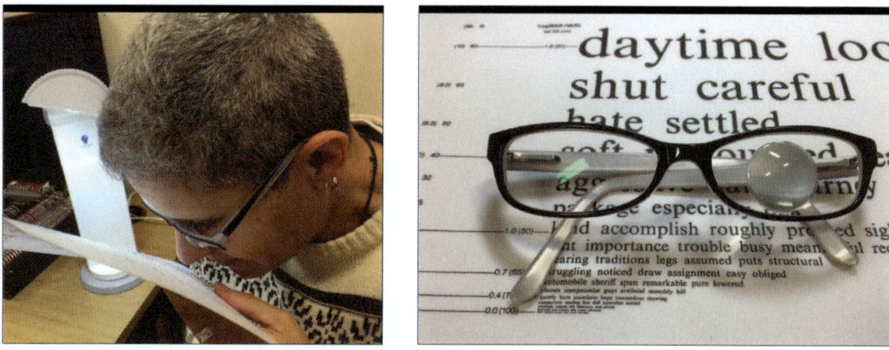

Figure 7.3 Alev has a +36D self adhesive Univision bifocal lens from *Eschenbach* mounted onto the front surface of her habitual distance prescription. The ultra-light, 22mm diameter button weights 1g and therefore offers negligible increase in spectacle weight and takes little time to assemble.

Multi-order diffractive lenses

Eschenbach's multi-order diffractive (MOD) lenses are covered in Chapter 6. In summary, these diffractive aspheric spectacle lenses are thin and lightweight with excellent visual performance and are not to be confused with the poor-quality optics produced by Fresnel 'sheet' magnifiers. The pre-ordered lenses have the same symmetrical shape and therefore may be mounted into either eye of an accompanying branded half eye frame whilst the patient is waiting. A frosted lens is placed in the fellow eye (Figure 7.4)

Compound lenses or lens systems

Compound lenses or lens systems combine two or more lenses together. The combination of lenses may be housed in a carrier mounted onto the patient's spectacle creating levels of magnification as high as 20x or more. They are often mistaken for telescopes; however, this is not the case as there may be minimal visible space between the two lenses. Figure 7.2 (centre), consists of an aplanatic doublet, previously described in Chapter 6. The purpose of the compound lens system is to achieve higher levels of magnification without the significant aberrational effect than would occur with a high-powered single vision lens. Compound lens systems are often used in the eyepiece and objectives of telescopes (Chapter 8).

Figure 7.4 The patient is using *Eschenbach's* half eye frame into which a multi-order diffractive (MOD) lens is providing 3x magnification (+12D) for one eye. The fellow eye is frosted. Both lenses are symmetrical and interchangeable so that the spectacle magnifier can be made up during the consultation from a bank of lens powers. The patient gains additional working distance by placing the half eye frame further down her nose. Total combined weight is just 20g.

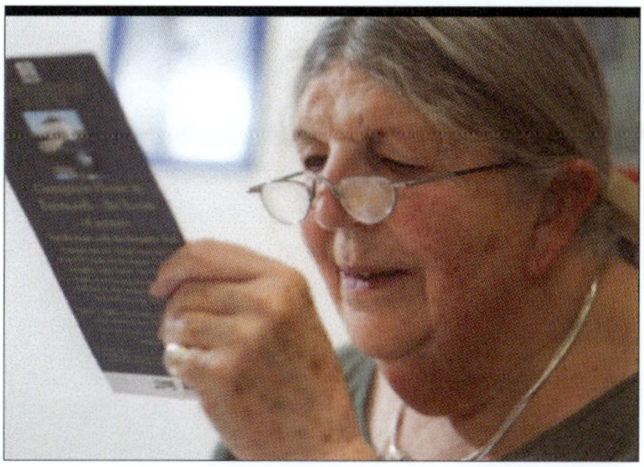

Clip-on solutions (monocular and binocular)

Additional plus lenses may be clipped over or onto the patient's current spectacle correction when required. Many designs include a hinge so that the lens may be flipped up out of the way when not required. These removable lenses tend to be available in lower powers binocularly and slightly higher powers monocularly. The clip-on lens seen in Figure 7.5 is mounted onto the end of a 5cm stem, which gives the patient that little extra working distance.

Figures 7.5 A) The patient is using a binocular clip-on lens (1.7x) from *Eschenbach* to read the newspaper. B) The patient is using a monocular 7x (+28D) clip-on over the spectacle lens of the right eye. As the lenses are mounted at the end of a stalk, the patient has the advantage of extending the overall working distance from the eye by a few more centimetres.

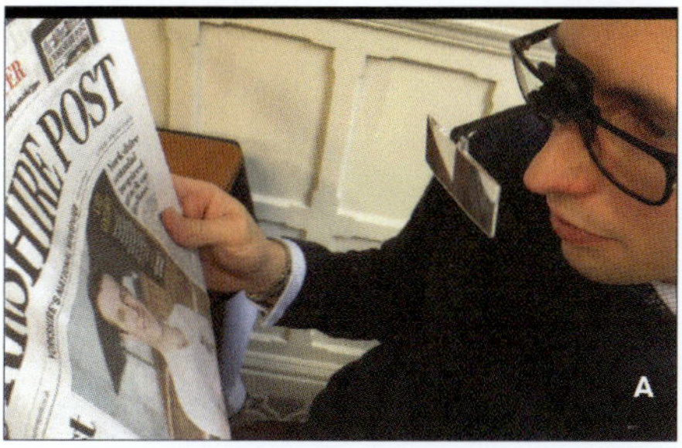

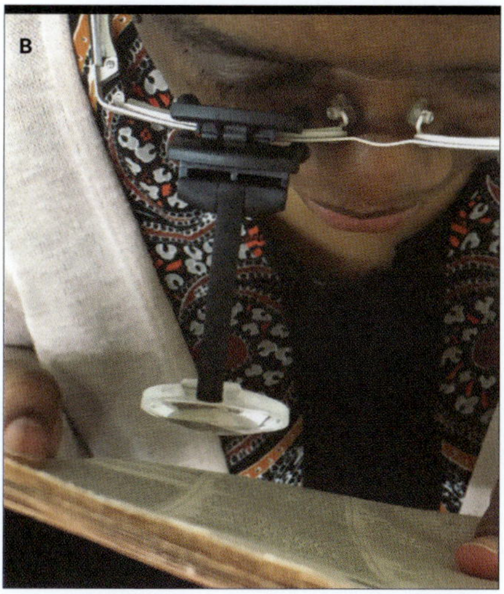

The need for occlusion

Most acquired conditions often affect each eye unequally so it is more usual to prescribe magnification to the better eye. However, some patients struggle with interfering distortion or diplopia and therefore it may be worth considering occlusion of the fellow eye to improve visual comfort. This is particularly relevant when the interference is from the previously dominant eye. This can be achieved by using a balancing, frosted, or opaque lens in the fellow eye. For those patients who do not like the appearance of a frosted lens, effective temporary solutions include the use of cotton wool pad, surgical tape, or an orthoptic medical eye patch (Figure 10.10, Chapter 10).

Range of available powers

The power range of spectacle magnifiers will vary across manufacturers due to the diverse range of lens forms, clip-ons or mounted additions available. However, the most significant factor limiting the range of practical magnification is the focal length of the plus lens used, which is the same regardless of lens form. Monocular solutions are available as either single or compound lenses up to approximately 20x (+80D) magnification. At this level of magnification, the patient will be holding text at a distance of only 1.25cm.

Maintaining cyl-correction

Most patients will require astigmatic errors over 1.50-2.00DC to be fully corrected. However, this is not a hard and fast rule and will vary according to the level of acuity the patient has and the nature of the impairment resulting from the underlying condition. For example, patients who have significant central loss, but who retain good peripheral vision, may still benefit from full cylindrical correction to assist with mobility.

Binocular spectacle magnifiers

When it is desirable or necessary to maintain binocularity, for example in the case of a patient with nystagmus (Chapter 4), the variety of spectacle based solutions is limited. Base-in prism or decentration will be required to avoid diplopia or confusion when the object is held at a shorter working distance due to the increase in convergence demand.[1] Most patients require base-in assistance when holding material consistently closer than approximately 25-20cm to maintain visual comfort. Binocular clip on units without base-in prism are therefore only available in the lower levels of magnification (Figure 7.5A).

Maintaining binocularity with prism incorporation

There are no hard and fast rules for how much prism or decentration is required for specific working distances; differences in interpupillary distances, accommodative convergence and heterophoria, for example, can vary considerably between patients. Therefore, if an individual spectacle order is to be made, practitioners may consider the following guidelines below, but to then recheck the amount of decentration or base-in prism for each patient on an individual basis.

Guidelines

For every dioptre [2-5] of focusing for near vision, whether by accommodation or lens addition, there is an associated one-meter angle of convergence. So, for any low vision patient viewing an object at 10 cm (e.g. +10.00D lens giving 2.5x magnification), 10 meter-angles of convergence will be required used to maintain binocular single vision. This value may be converted into prism dioptres by multiplying the interpupillary distance in centimetres by the meter-angle value.

To allow for the extra convergence, adequate decentration or base-in prism should be worked; a rule-of-thumb being '1 mm in decentration of bifocal segment for each dioptre of reading addition for each eye or, for single vision lenses, one prism dioptre base-in ground on lenses for each dioptre of reading addition in each eye.'

Example:

For a +10D reading addition, 10^{Δ} will be required in each eye.

Prismatic spectacles

'Ready-made' spectacles incorporating pre-determined base base-in prism to assist convergence are available from one or two manufacturers; the amount of prism calculated, however, is based upon the amount of plus power in the spectacles and therefore assumes that the patient is emmetropic or nearly so to begin with.

These 'prismatic spectacles' as they are often called, are available with powers ranging from approximately +4D to +16D with prism incorporation of approximately 4^{Δ} to 16^{Δ} base-in each eye respectively, with slight variation in prism values between manufacturers (Figures 7. 2 (bottom) and 7.6.

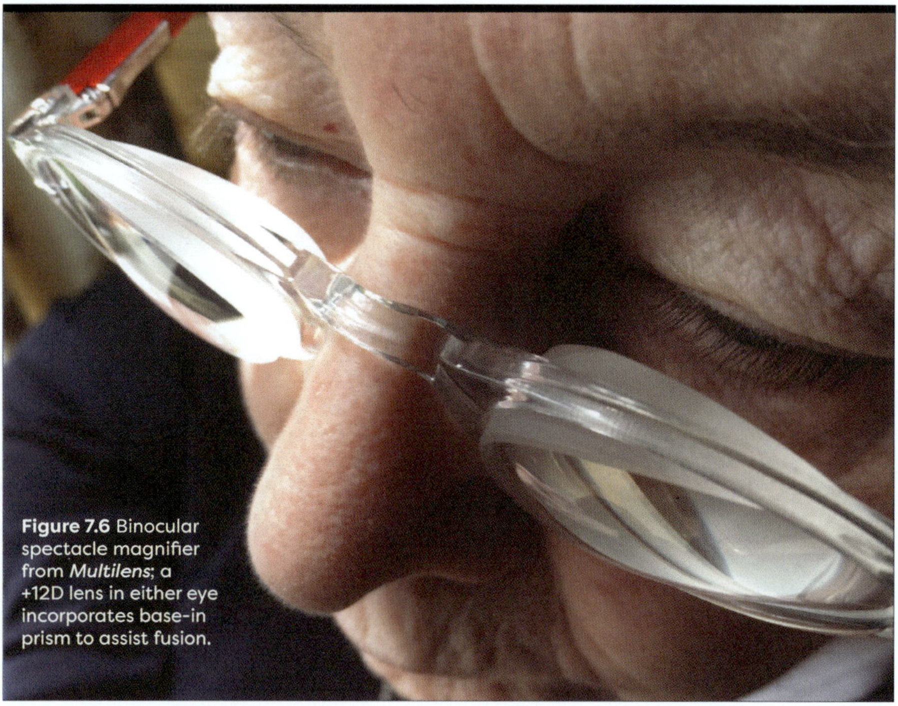

Figure 7.6 Binocular spectacle magnifier from *Multilens*; a +12D lens in either eye incorporates base-in prism to assist fusion.

Adapting to working close

Many older patients, who have spent a lifetime with a book on their lap, often find the closer working distance of higher-powered spectacle magnifiers difficult to achieve and maintain. On the other hand, young patients with a congenital visual impairment tend to have a higher success rate, achieving natural relative distance enlargement by holding text or objects close using strong accommodative effort. However, when accommodation begins to drop, those same patients may require a reading addition to maintain the same close working distance.[6]

Those with acquired visual impairment who do make the compromise often develop inventive ways of achieving and maintaining the shorter working distances including the use of reading stands, lap trays, wrap-round scarves, piles of cushions, to name but a few.

When working at very close distances, patients will need extra illumination. Miniature clip-on LED lights are available from several bookstores that can be attached onto the book. Alternatively, some are also available to clip onto the spectacles themselves.

Determining success

During the low vision assessment, establish the patient's response to the shorter working distance. If possible, use a Halberg clip over the patient's habitual reading prescription. This gives the patient the opportunity to make direct comparisons and thus appreciate the difference in both the effect of magnification and the new working distance. This may be more difficult to achieve when using a trial frame. In addition, measure the new working distance and write it down for the patient to remember.

However, an ability to demonstrate the success of a spectacle magnifier in a consulting room does not necessarily translate into use in the patient's favourite armchair. Be alert to this possibility and warn patients of the importance of remembering to move objects into the appropriate position.

Comparison with a telescope unit

If a patient is struggling with the shorter working distance of the spectacle magnifier but is still keen to find a hands-free solution, then the similar powered spectacle mounted telescope will offer the patient a longer working distance, albeit with a more restricted field of view:

Example:

A Galilean 2.5x distance unit with an addition +8D end cap will offer 5x magnification for near at a working distance of 12.5cms. The equivalent 5x spectacle magnifier will consist of a +20D lens with a working distance of 5cm. However, although the telescope in this example offers over twice the working distance, it has a more restricted field of view of 11°.

The field of view of the spectacle magnifier is dependent upon the diameter of the lens or lens system used and is thus less restrictive than looking down the barrel of a telescope.

References

1. Bither PP. Determining the convergence demand for a patient who reads at a close working distance. Am J Optom Physiol Opt. 1987;64(5):355–60.
2. Fonda GE. Designing half-eye binocular spectacle magnifiers. Surv Ophthalmol. 1991;36(2):149–54.
3. Katz M. Convergence demands by spectacle magnifiers. Vol. 73, Optometry & Vision Science. 1996. p. 540–5.
4. Bailey I. Centering high-addition spectacle lenses. Optom Mon. 1979;(70):523–7.
5. Bailey I. Magnification for near vision. Optom Mon. 1980;(71:73-6).
6. Leat SJ, Mohr A. Accommodative response in pre-presbyopes with visual impairment and its clinical implications. Investig Ophthalmol Vis Sci. 2007 Aug 1;48(8):3888–96.

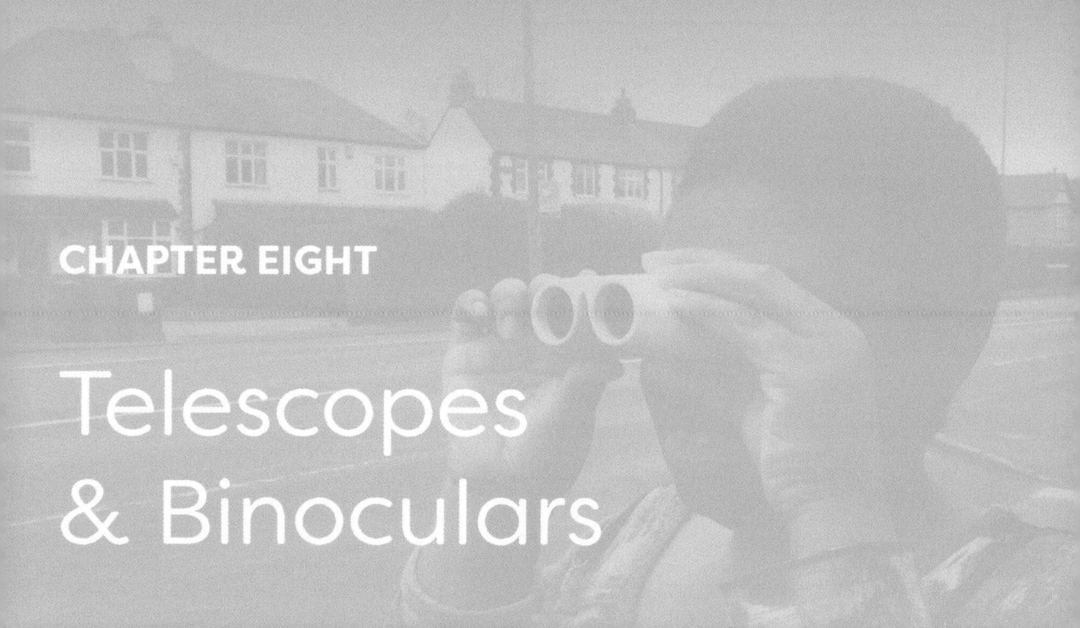

CHAPTER EIGHT

Telescopes & Binoculars

“The demands of everyday living tasks and maintaining employment for a person with a visual impairment are complex and manifold. The challenges presented are frequently demanding and sometimes can only be met by improvisation and combination of products from different sources, sometimes applied differently to the original design intention.”

Kevin McNally FBDO (Hons) LVA BSc (Hons) MCOptom
Kettering General and Hinchingbrooke NHS trusts

Telescopes & Binoculars

Introduction

There is an upward trend for patients to use electronic devices or smart phone applications offering distance or near magnification. There is also a growing number of GPS led navigation applications offering assistance to people with visual impairement when traveling on foot or using public transport. However, telescopes and binoculars are still a fundamental method of magnifying distance and intermediate objects. For near magnification tasks, spectacle-mounted telescopes offer a hands-free solution with a longer working distance compared to the equivalent spectacle lens magnifier of similar power. For example in Figure 8.1, the patient is using a 2.1x clip-on binocular telescope to read a newspaper at a comfortable working distance of 35cm. In comparison, a 2x (+8D) spectacle magnifier would have a working distance of 12.5cm, being the focal length of the additional plus lens used.

Commonly reported distance or intermediate tasks

A list of commonly reported distance tasks is outlined in Chapter 2. Many distance and intermediate tasks such as seeing the edges of kerbs and steps, or being able to cross the road, may not be solved with distance magnification. Patients with these needs are referred for mobility interventions by rehabilitation teams. However, the list below of commonly reported distance tasks may indeed benefit from the use of a telescopic aid:

- Watching television, viewing subtitles
- Identifying buses/bus numbers
- Scoreboards at sporting events
- Travelling on the underground

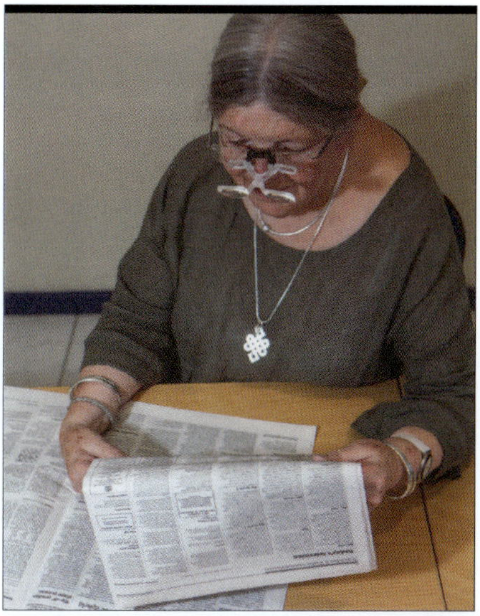

Figure 8.1 The patient is wearing a 2.1x clip-on Galilean telescope by *Eschenbach* offering a hands-free view at 35cm. The unit adds just 23g of additional weight and has an 18^0 wide binocular field of view. The unit may be flipped up, or slipped off the spectacles when not required

- Train indicator boards
- Street names
- Shopping aisles in the supermarket
- Galleries and museums
- Theatre / cinema outings
- Playing Bridge
- Reading music
- Notice boards, bus timetables

Distance magnification

There are essentially only a few fundamental ways in which a patient can make the appearance of distance placed objects appear larger.

- Move closer to the object
- Use a telescope (or binocular)
- Capture an image digitally, enlarge or enhance and reproduce it on screen such as a, smartphone or a head-mounted display unit (HMD).

The effect of moving closer to the object

By decreasing the viewing distance and moving in closer to the object, the retinal image size will increase (relative distance magnification). This may not always be practical to do.

The retinal image size of a patient sitting at 1m from a television screen will be the same as sitting at a 3m viewing distance and wearing a 3x telescope. Eyecare practitioners regularly tell patients to sit closer to the television to achieve magnification of the screen to avoid the restricted field of view looking through a telescopic device. However, a large majority of our older patients, especially those with a significant loss of acuity, are unwilling to alter the position of furniture within their homes. Fear of falling over repositioned items or the need to adapt to significant change is frequently met with a degree of reluctance and is worth bearing in mind when making such a suggestion. Furthermore, it is not uncommon to find that a patient has been previously avoiding sitting so close to a television for fear of causing harm to his or her eyesight.

If a patient is willing to sit significantly closer to the object then in some cases a change in spectacle prescription may also be useful. A patient who sits at a distance of 1m from a television set, for example, may benefit from an additional +1.00D addition to their distance correction.

Estimating magnification

All distance devices that are telescopic in nature, exploit angular magnification. Estimating magnification required for distance tasks is relatively straightforward and prescribing more so due to a relatively small range of available telescopic devices designed specifically for people with a visual impairment.

Once the patient's distance refraction has been determined, then estimating the amount of magnification required to see an object is a simple ratio comparison between the patient's current acuity and the size of the object that he or she wishes to view. Hence, if a patient's distance acuity is 6/60, then theoretically they should require 10× magnification to achieve 6/6 (i.e. comparing denominator values, 60÷6). Similarly, if a patient's distance acuity is 6/36 then 4x magnification should improve their acuity close to 6/9 (comparing denominator values 36÷9). In reality however, no two patients behave the same way and therefore practitioners can use these calculations merely as a guide. In addition, most patients will not have the need to obtain 6/6 acuity with a telescope. It is more common to aim for an acuity of approximately 6/12-6/9 for the majority of day-to-day distance tasks. When deciding between two levels of magnification, for example, between a 4x and a 6x telescope, first-time users may opt for the weaker of the two magnification devices that offers a better field of view and greater image stability. More experienced telescopic users may then opt for a higher level of magnification when they have become more proficient at using a device.

The above examples are useful when estimating magnification using Snellen notation. For those practitioners who use logMAR charts, then the estimated magnification is a simple product of the number of successive lines on a logMAR chart, with the difference in magnification between each line being 1.26x. This is outlined in Table 8.1.

Example:

The magnification required to improve a patient's distance acuity from 6/60 (logMAR 1.00) to 6/12 is 5x magnification. This is the same as improving a patient's logMAR acuity from 1.0 to 0.3, a difference of 7 lines of a logMAR chart, which is also difference of 5x magnification.

Table 8.1 Magnification factor between successive lines of logMAR acuity.

Lines of improvement in logMAR	Magnification required
1	1.26x
2	1.6x
3	2x
4	2.5x
5	3.2x
6	4x
7	5x
8	6.4x
9	8x
10	10x

History of telescopes

In 1608, two Flemish spectacle-makers, Hans Lippershey and Jacob Metius independently of each other applied for patents for the first refracting telescope. News of these new devices, described "for seeing things far away as if they were nearby," soon reached Galileo Galilei who then worked out the principles for himself, building his own 8x version in 1609. Galileo was subsequently accredited as the first to use a telescope to observe the stars. Johannes Kepler improved the design further, building his own device in 1610.

The history of using telescopes as an aid to low vision is scant. Whether visually impaired or not, telescopes have been used to magnify distant objects that have been difficult to see, therefore their use as a low vision aid has developed naturally over time. It was not until the 1950's, however, that the provision of telescopes as an aid to those with a visual impairment, became a professional service, with Charles Keeler being one of the more notable members of the optical profession to develop this area of clinical practice.[1]

The original stargazing telescopes built by Galileo and Kepler, however were long, as a result of, amongst a number of factors, the use of relatively low-powered lenses, which were ground by hand. By using higher-powered lenses with significantly shorter focal lengths, telescopes used for low vision are now shorter in length and thus more compact and portable than their predecessors. Optical performance is further improved with the use of high quality lenses and coatings that together produce clearer, brighter images.

The principles of telescope designs

All telescopic low vision aids are based upon two principal designs of distance telescopes, the Galilean and the Keplerian telescope. The original telescopes were afocal, being designed to study the stars from which incident light reaching the telescope would have zero vergence.

In reality, when a telescope is used as a low vision aid, the majority of objects that a person with visual impairement needs to be able to view will not be at infinity. Commonly reported tasks include, for example, viewing train indicator boards, watching the television or reading music when placed on a music stand. At distances closer than infinity, incident vergence entering the telescopic system is no longer zero and must now be corrected to focus the image upon the retina. Secondly, eyes tend not to be emmetropic and therefore for the most part, the basic afocal telescope will require modification. Any modification will ultimately have an effect on the telescope design and resultant magnification.

Telescopic magnification

A telescope is constructed by an objective lens at the far end of the tube (also known as the entrance pupil) and the eyepiece lens, which is closest to the user's eye. To achieve magnification (M_{tel}), the eyepiece lens (Fe) must always be the stronger in power:

$$M_{tel} = -Fe/Fo$$

In a Galilean system, the eyepiece is a concave lens and the objective lens (Fo) is convex. The resultant magnification of the telescope is positive, indicating that the image is erect. When viewing an object at infinity, the length of the telescope (t) is calculated as the sum of the focal lengths of both the objective and eyepiece lenses (Figure 8.2).

Galilean telescope worked example:

Magnification (M_{tel})

Fe	= -40D
Fo	= +20D
M_{tel}	= - (-40)/20
M_{tel}	= x2

Telescope length (t):

t	= fe' + fo'
t	= (-25) + (+50)
t	= 25mm

In a Keplerian system, the eyepiece (Fe) is a convex lens and thus positive in power. The image viewed is now inverted and laterally reversed (Figure 8.3). This also indicated by the negative sign on the magnification calculation in the following example.

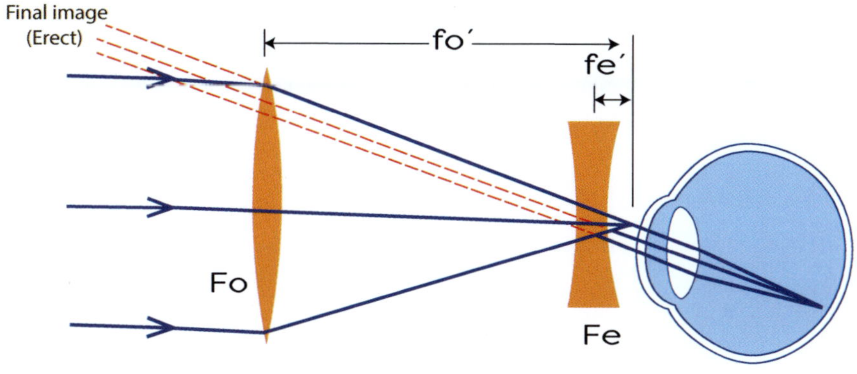

Figure 8.2
The Galilean telescope is viewing light from a distant object.
The image produced is erect.
Eyepiece Fe, Objective Fo,
Focal length of eyepiece fe', Focal length of objective fo', telescope length, t

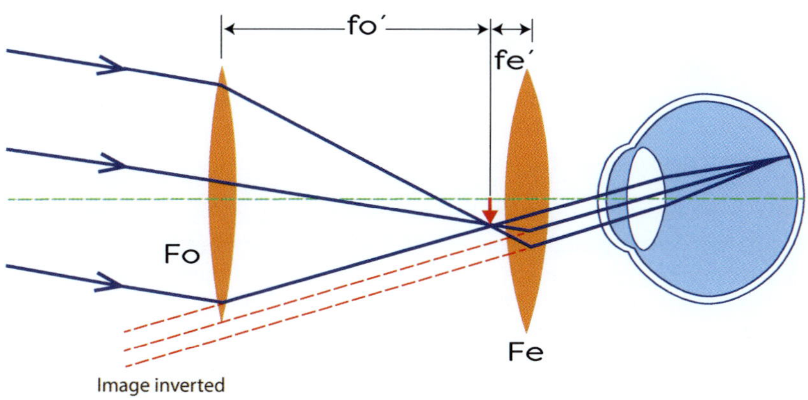

Figure 8.3
The Keplerian telescope is viewing light from a distant object.
The image produced is inverted and laterally reversed.
Eyepiece Fe, Objective Fo,
Focal length of eyepiece fe, Focal length of objective fo,

Keplerian telescope worked example:

Magnification (M_{tel})	
Fe	= +40D
Fo	= +20D
M_{tel}	= - 40/20
M_{tel}	= x-2
Telescope length:	
t	= fe' + fo'
t	= (+25) + (+50)
t	= 75mm

The Kepler design will therefore be longer in length compared to the Galilean telescope of equivalent magnification. From the above equation it also follows that the higher the power of the lenses incorporated within the unit, the shorter the focal lengths and thus the shorter the tube length. Consequently, compound lens systems (consisting of two or more lenses) are often used to increase overall power of the eyepiece and objective 'lenses' and thus create a more compact unit. However, the combination of more than one lens in a compound lens system has the disadvantage of increasing the number of lens surfaces. Coatings that are then added to compensate for the consequence of increased aberrations will ultimately push up the cost of the device.

Prism erecting systems

In Kepler's design the image of the stars was inverted and laterally reversed, but it was not until Ignazio Porro in 1854, over 200 years since Galileo and Kepler's designs, that a prism erecting system was developed to place the image the 'right way up.' In the 1890's the Carl Zeiss Foundation, with the help of Ernst Abbe and Mortiz Hensoldt refined Porro's prism erecting system, further developing new prism erecting systems, known as roof prisms and incorporating them into their own optical devices.

Incorporating a prism within the telescope adds weight and depending upon the type of prism or prism system used, will impact upon the physical design of the telescope and image quality. The incorporation of a double Porro prism system will result in a bulkier unit compared to a telescope containing a roof prism system. This is because a Porro prism system alters the line of sight, with the added effect of reducing the overall length of the tube (Figure 8.4). Incorporation of a roof prism system, of which there are several designs, creates a straight optical light path and thus a slimmer, longer unit (Figure 8.5). The Porro prism system benefits from total internal reflection across its surfaces, whereas some roof prisms require coated surfaces to improve reflectivity.

Entrance and exit pupils

Light enters the telescope through the objective lens, also known as the entrance pupil. The telescope lens system concentrates the light gathered by the objective into a beam, which then leaves the telescope through the exit pupil, a point that does not correspond with the eyepiece lens. In the Galilean system the exit pupil appears within, or internal to the telescope system and in the Keplerian telescope the exit pupil is external and virtual to the system, i.e. it appears between the eye and the eyepiece as seen in Figure 8.6.

Telescopes and binoculars are described in terms of their magnification and objective lens diameter. For example, an 8 x 20 unit has a magnification (M_{tel}) of 8x and an objective lens diameter of 20mm. Larger diameter objectives will collect more light resulting in a brighter, better quality image. The field of view of a device marginally increases with the diameter of the objective. Figure 8.7 shows three 8x telescopes used as low vision devices, each with increasing diameter of objective lenses. In producing the same level of magnification in each device, the units that contain larger diameter lenses often use lower powered lens powers, which will result in larger and longer telescope units.

From a practical point of view, the patient will achieve the best field of view and the brightest image through a telescope when the exit pupil is the same size as the patient's own 'entrance' pupil. If the telescope exit pupil is larger than the patient's pupil then the excess light is wasted. Patient's are also encouraged to hold the telescope as close to the eye as possible; those who have small pupils may need assistance to locate the telescope's exit pupil, especially when using a Keplerian device as the exit pupil is so much smaller than that found in a Galilean design. A rubberised eyepiece cup, present on the end of a Keplerian telescope, assists patients in locating the exit pupil as it allows the patient to rest the telescope within the orbit and thus closer to the eye. For spectacle wearers, the eyepiece cup may then be folded back,allowing a protective, rubberised end to come into contact with the spectacle lenses and thus bring the exit pupil closer to the patient's eye (Figure 8.8).

Figure 8.4 Two Porro prisms are placed at right angles to each other within the barrel of the telescope to produce an image that is erect and laterally corrected. The light path is 'folded' resulting in the shorter, but bulkier unit

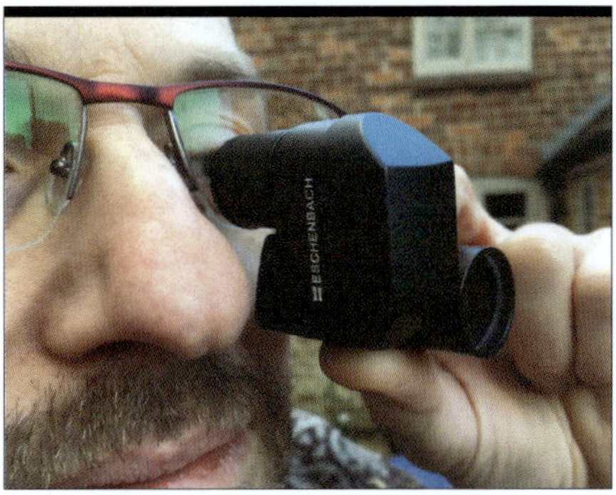

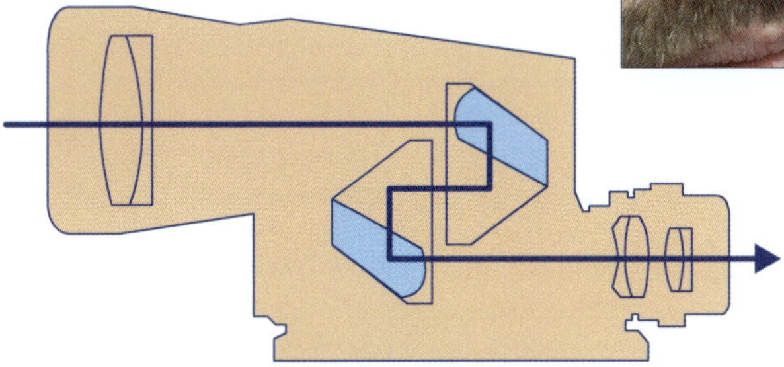

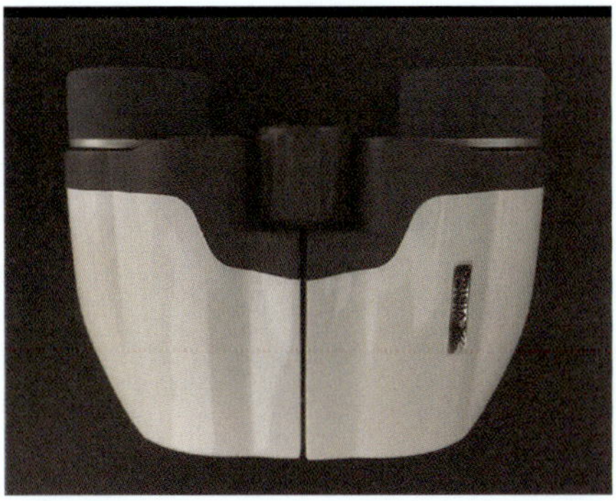

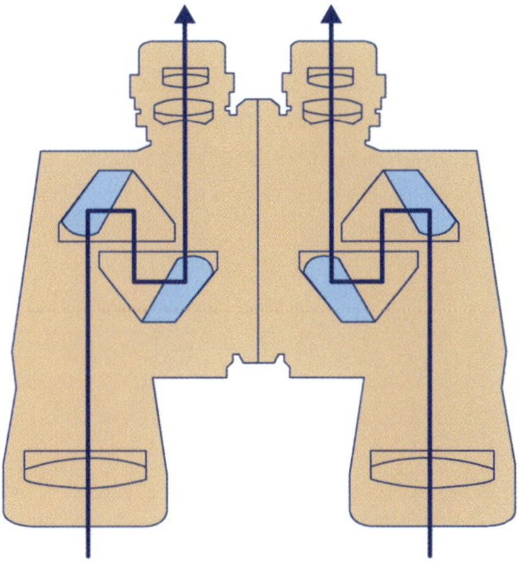

Figure 8.5 A roof prism system is placed within the barrel of the Keplerian telescope which produces a straight optical light path.

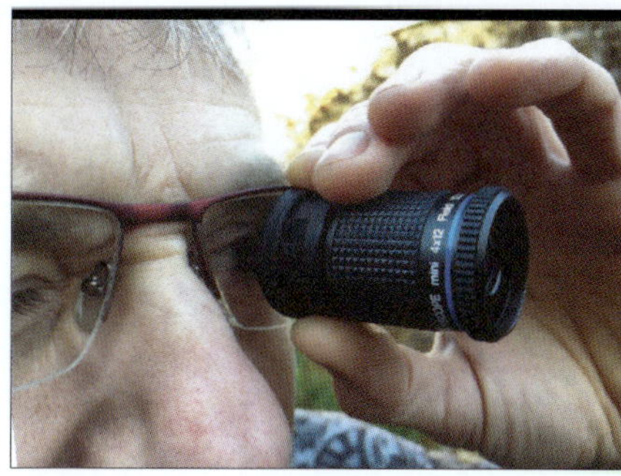

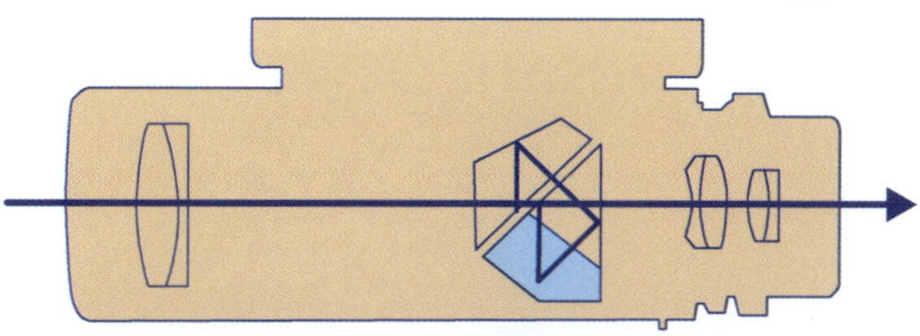

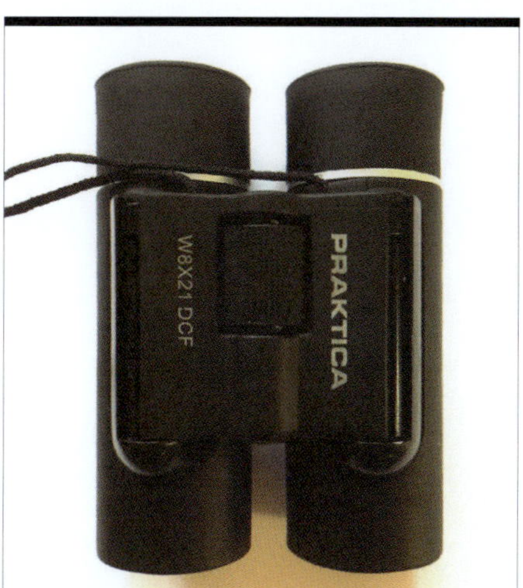

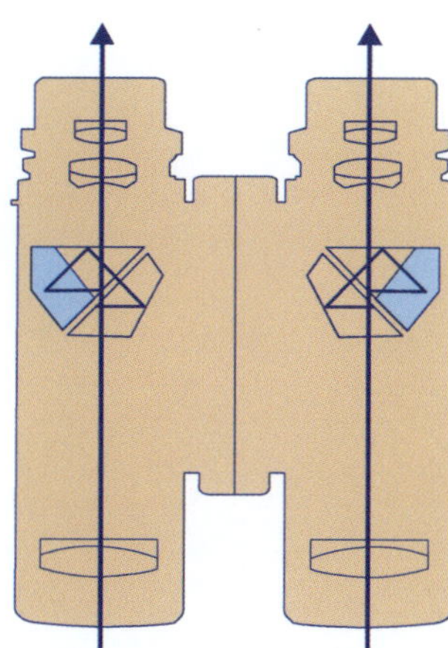

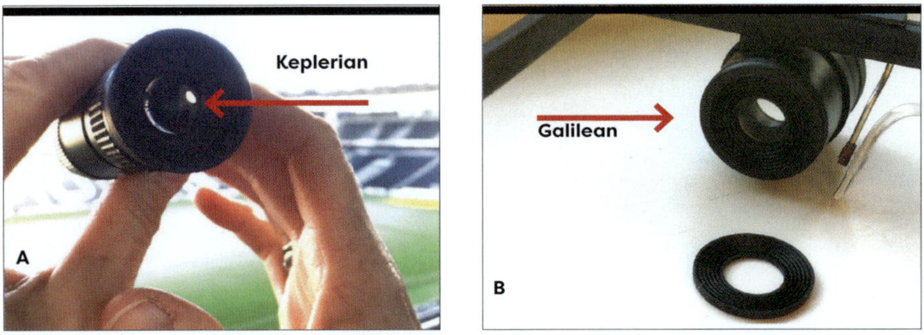

Figure 8.6 The smaller exit pupil of the Keplerian telescope (A) is closer to the patient's own pupil and is external to the barrel of the device. The Galilean exit pupil (B) is larger and further away from the eye and is contained within the barrel of the device. The additional auxiliary lens may be glazed with the patient's distance correction and added to the eyepiece.

Figure 8.7 Three 8x telescopes each with decreasing objective diameter (32, 25 and 20mm from left to right) which has a significant impact upon the size of the telescope

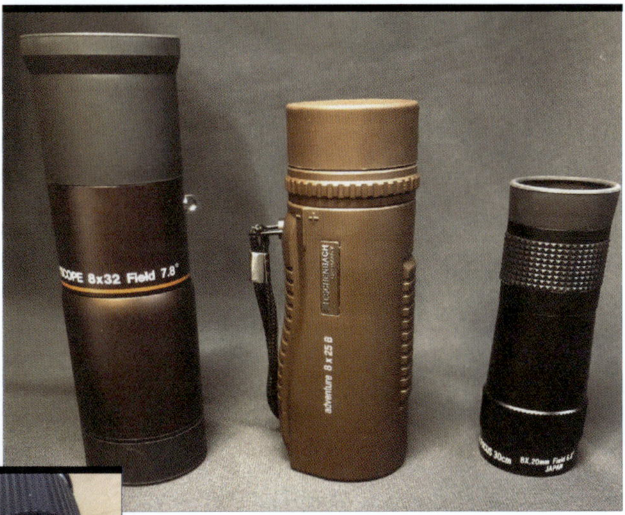

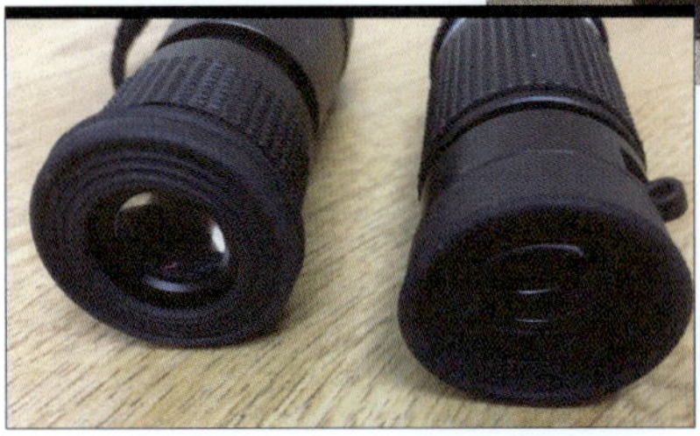

Figure 8.8 The rubberised eyecup of the telescope may be folded back allowing the telescope to be placed on the anterior lens surface

Modifications

Using a telescope at a finite distance

Vergence is amplified, or magnified, when it passes through a telescope system. The calculation of vergence amplification is complex,[2] however an approximate working formula is described below:[3]

$$\text{emergent vergence} = (M_{tel})^2 \times \text{incident vergence}$$

Therefore, if an 8x afocal distance monocular were used to view a train indicator board at a distance of 3m, then the incident vergence from the target entering the telescope would be -0.3D. Thus:

$$\begin{aligned}\text{emergent vergence} &= (M_{tel})^2 \times \text{incident vergence}\\ &= (8)^2 \times -0.3\text{D}\\ &= -19.2\text{D}\end{aligned}$$

Even at distance of 3m a patient using an 8x telescope would require a large degree of accommodation (19.2D) to focus the target. To compensate for this amplification effect, a number of modifications can be made to the telescope:

Altering the separation between eyepiece and objective.

Incident vergence from a near object may be corrected as it travels through the telescope by increasing the separation between both the eyepiece and objective lenses (Figure 8.9). The telescope itself is now focused on a finitely placed object and as such is now described as a **focal** telescope. Altering the separation between the eyepiece and objective lenses in adjustable focus devices has the added advantage of being able to compensate for a small degree of spherical refractive error.

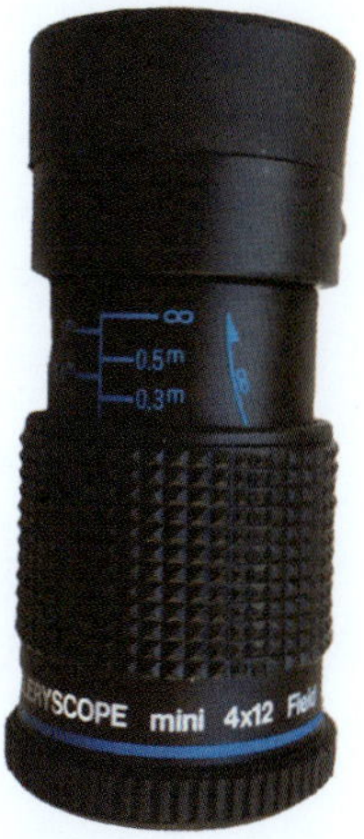

Figure 8.9 By increasing the telescope length, the patient can focus this 4x monocular as close as 23cm

However, variable focus telescopes and binoculars require the use of both hands to focus the image, whereas the non-adjustable telescope that the patient is using in Figure 8.10 only requires the use of one hand.

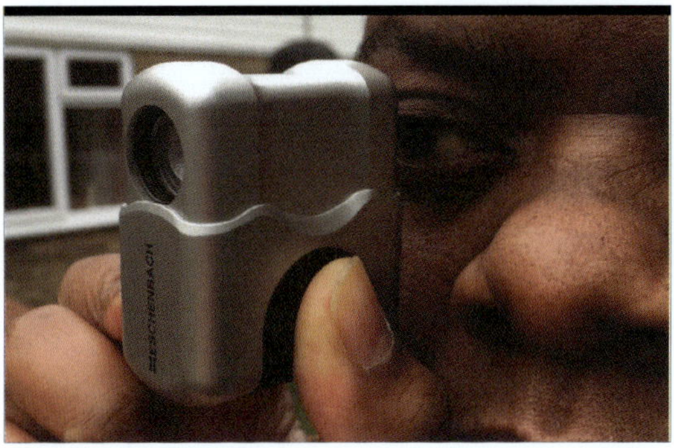

Figure 8.10 This simple 4x unit is in focus from 4m to infinity and requires no focus. This device is often favoured by children and by patients who struggle with adjustable devices or who only have the use of one hand. This patient should be encouraged to bring the telescope closer to her eye to achieve the best field of view

Adding an end cap

Vergence may be corrected before it enters the telescope by adding a simple plus lens 'end cap' to the objective. This method is used, for example, with spectacle mounted telescopes such as those seen in Figure 8.11 where a distance unit is mounted onto the patient's spectacles and an additional end cap may be added converting the telescope for use at near. The total magnification of the device when used at near will be the product of the magnification provided by both the distance unit (M_{tel}) and the reading cap (M_{cap}). The working distance of the object or reading material should then be held at the focal length of the end cap. A summary is presented is Table 8.2.

Worked example 1:

If a 2.2x distance Galilean spectacle-mounted telescope is used to view an object at 10cm, an end cap of +10D will neutralise the -10D incident vergence entering the telescope. The power of the end-cap will have an effect on the overall magnification of the system:

Magnification of telescope (M_{tel}) = 2.2x

Magnification of the end cap (M_{cap}) = (F/4) = 10/4 = 2.5x

Total magnification at near (M_{tel} x M_{cap}) = (2.2 x 2.5) = 5.5x

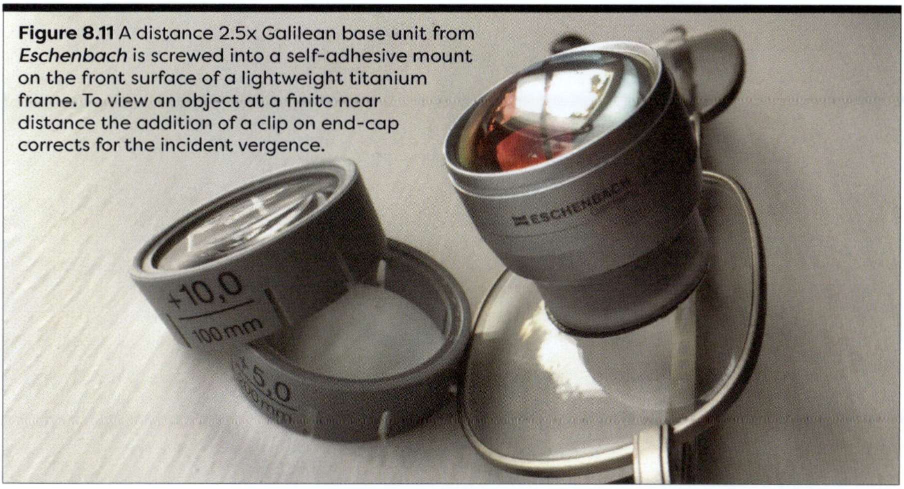

Figure 8.11 A distance 2.5x Galilean base unit from *Eschenbach* is screwed into a self-adhesive mount on the front surface of a lightweight titanium frame. To view an object at a finite near distance the addition of a clip on end-cap corrects for the incident vergence.

The main purpose of using a telescope for near is to provide a hands free solution with an extended working distance compared to a spectacle lens magnifier offering the same level of magnification. In worked example 2, if a patient needs 5x magnification for near, then the equivalent spectacle lens magnifier power would be a +20D lens (M=F/4) with a focal length working distance of 5cm.

The 5x telescope example offers over twice the working distance of the spectacle lens magnifier. However at the higher powers of magnification of 8-10x or more, the difference in working distance between the telescope and spectacle lens magnifier becomes significantly less.

Worked example 2:

A patient requires a 5x spectacle-mounted telescope for use at near:

If the Galilean spectacle mounted distance unit has a magnification (M_{tel}) of 2.5x, then the patient would require 5x/2.5x = 2x magnification in the end cap to achieve this.

The power of the end cap will therefore need to be +8.00D (M_{cap}=F/4). The working distance that the patient will need to hold the object will be the focal length of the end cap, in this case 12.5cm.

Table 8.2 Comparison of two *Eschenbach* Galilean distance telescopic units and the effect of adding an end cap to magnification and working distance, with a comparison of the working distance (WD) of an equivalent spectacle lens magnifier[4]

Cap Power 6g	Combined magnification of telescope unit +end cap		Working Distance (mm)	
	Galilei 2.2x Distance Unit Field of View 14°, 16g, Hard coat	Galilei 2.5x Distance Unit Field of View 13°, 11g MAR Coat	Telescope + end cap	Comparable Spectacle lens magnifier
Cap +3D Available binoc. in 2.2x unit	1.65x	1.9x	330mm	1.75x /+7D = 143mm
Cap +4D Available binoc. in 2.2x unit	2.2x	2.5x	250mm	2.5x /+10D = 100mm
Cap +5D Available binoc. in 2.2x unit	2.75x	3.15x	200mm	3x /+12D = 83mm
Cap +6D monoc. only	3.3x	3.75x	167mm	3.5x /+14D = 71mm
Cap +8D monoc. only	4.4x	5.0x	125mm	5x /+20D = 50mm
Cap +10D monoc. only	5.5x	6.25x	100mm	6x /+24D = 42mm
Cap +12D monoc. only	6.6x	7.5x	83mm	7x /+28D = 36mm
Cap +16D monoc. only	8.8x	10.0x	63mm	9x /+36D = 28mm 10x /+40D = 25mm

Correcting for refractive error

Mountings, clips and carriers

When a patient needs their full distance spectacle correction in place, a telescope may then be screwed into a simple, self-adhesive carrier mounted on the front surface of the spectacle lens as seen in Figure 8.11. These adhesive mounts significantly reduce chair time and cost compared to previous carriers that required cementing onto the spectacle lens by a prescription house. Alternatively, some telescope designs may utilize a simple clip so that the telescope may be removed or flipped up out of the way when not required, such as that seen in Figure 8.1.

With some designs however, the patient's spectacle correction may be glazed into a small auxiliary lens unit that may then be clipped directly over the telescope's eyepiece lens (Figure 8.6B). This is particularly useful for those patients who have a significant cylindrical error.

Adjustable focus and effect upon magnification

Adjustable telescopes and binoculars are not only able to compensate for the incident vergence of near objects as outlined above, but will also go some way to correct for a patient's spherical refractive error. For example, the simple Galilean designed "TV glasses" seen in Figure 8.12, are able to compensate for spherical refractive error of up to ±3.00DS.

Figure 8.12 Binocular 'television glasses' from *Eschenbach* offering 2.1x magnification. The unit is only 49g in weight and the adjustable cogs compensate from approx. -3.00D to +3.00D of spherical spectacle error. The negative eye piece lenses identify this unit as a Galilean telescope.

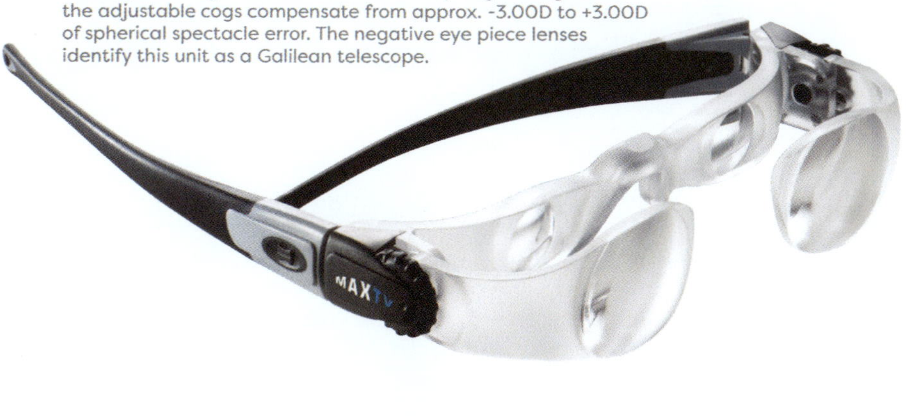

When a patient with a significant degree of ametropia uses a device without his or her spectacles, there will be a change in the level of magnification achieved through the device:

Galilean telescope worked example:

Fe	=	-40D
Fo	=	+20D
M	=	-Fe/Fo
	=	2x
Telescope length (t)	=	fe' + fo'
	=	(-25) + (50)
	=	25 mm

If a -5D myope were to use the above telescope, he would theoretically 'borrow' 5D from the -40D eyepiece, hypothetically changing it to a -35D eyepiece lens:

Fe	=	-35D
Fo	=	+20D
M	=	1.75x
t	=	21.4 mm

If the above Galilean telescope is used again by a +5D hypermetrope, then theoretically his uncorrected hyperopia is 'added' to the eyepiece:

Fe	=	-45D
Fo	=	+20D
M	=	2.25x
t	=	27.7 mm

A myope will therefore achieve less magnification from using a Galilean telescope and will shorten the tube length, whereas the hypermetrope will achieve more magnification and will extend the tube length when using the same telescope. The reverse is true in both cases when using a Keplerian design. In practical terms however, the above change in magnification is relatively small. Also, higher degrees of refractive error (beyond approximately ±4.00DS for most manufacturers) may not be corrected in this way due to the restrictions in altering the tube lengths.

Telescopes for mobility

Telescopes have been in use for some by patients to provide magnification whilst mobile, for example to magnify station train timetables, locating street signs or assisting navigation around the supermarket aisles. The majority of devices used for this purpose are hand held and are often hung around the neck on a cord or carried within a bag or pocket. However the telescope seen in Figure 8.13, known as a BiOptic, has been designed to sit permanently on the patient's distance correction, providing more timely magnification when required.

By incorporating a series of internal mirrors within a lightweight Keplerian telescope, the BiOptic unit can be mounted across the spectacles rather than projecting outwards. The single eyepiece lens is placed superior to the

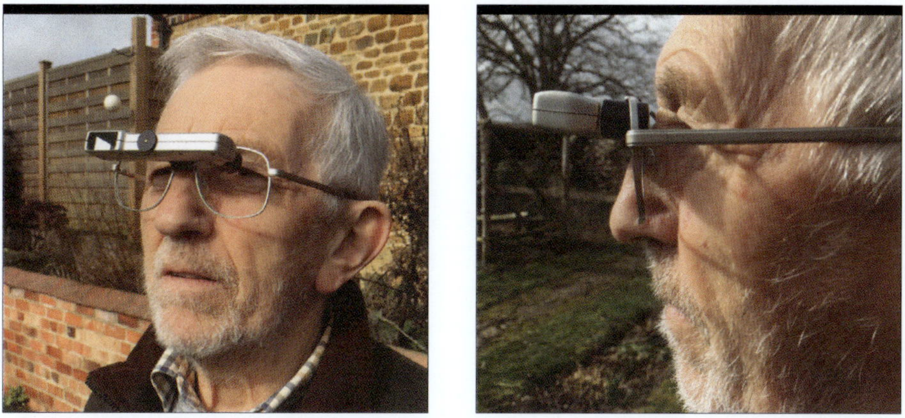

Figure 8.13 This 26g adjustable BiOptic unit from *Ocutech* is mounted superior to the line of sight by 10°. The patient can walk around freely and then drop his head when stationary to view a distant object when required. The unit compensates for +/-12D of spherical refractive error and up to 3.00DC of cylindrical error

visual axis and is angled slightly upwards by approximately 10°. The frame is glazed with the patient's habitual correction for general viewing and when magnification is required, the patient drops his head to look through the telescope. This type of telescope boasts a range of working distances from infinity to 25cm and has been successfully used for intermediate tasks such as reading music and playing bridge. The telescope is comfortable to wear for long periods of time and several users wear their unit whilst out of doors to improve navigation and mobility.

The BiOptic telescope extends the range of use of a spectacle mounted telescope for distance, intermediate and near working distances whilst the patient retains the advantage of remaining mobile. In a selected number of countries and US states, BiOptics have been approved for driving under a restricted licence.

Summary

Telescopes and binoculars are used by all age groups as mobility aids, and as magnification devices offering magnification for the full range of object distances ranging from infinity to near. This makes them the most versatile of low vision aids and an indispensible tool to improve independence and daily living tasks.

References

1. Keeler C. Visual aids for the pathological eye; excluding contact lenses. Trans Ophthalmol Soc United Kingdom. 1956;76:605–14.
2. Fried AN. Telescopes, light, vergence and accommodation. Am J Optom Physiol Opt. 1977;54(6):365–73.
3. Bailey I. New method for determining the magnifying power of telescopes. Am J Optom Physiol Opt. 1978;55(3):203–7.
4. Eschenbach. Eschenbach product catalogue [Internet]. [cited 2017 Nov 5]. Available from: http://www.eschenbach-sehhilfen.com

CHAPTER NINE

Electronic Magnification & Image Enhancement

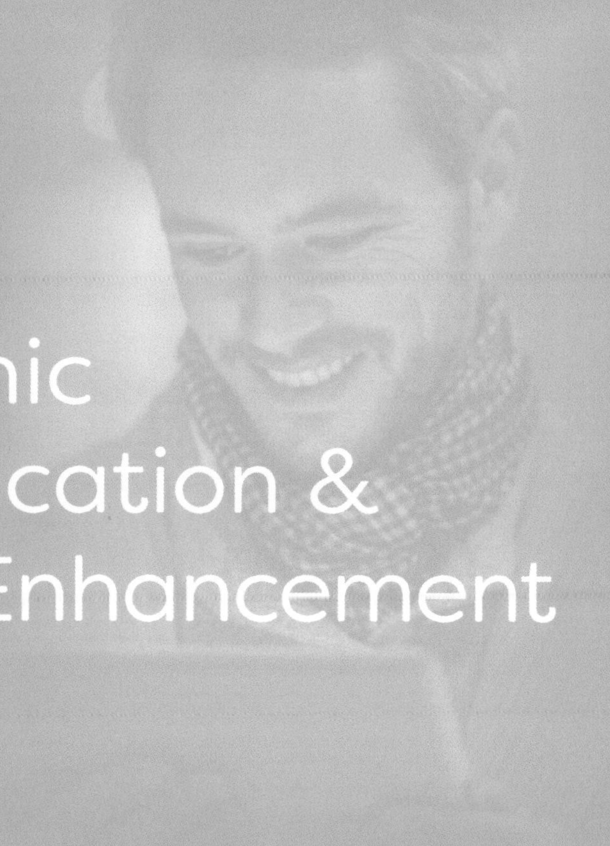

> "The cultural acceptability of handheld electronic devices has removed many of the concerns from patients with a visual impairment, about the use of digital magnifiers in social settings."

Dr Annette Parkinson PhD MCOptom Prof Cert LV FHEA
School of Optometry and Vision Science, Bradford,

Electronic Magnification & Image Enhancement

Introduction

At present, optical low vision aids such as hand or stand magnifiers, remain the device of preference offered by most low vision practitioners and low vision services. However, we are all aware that an increasing number of our patients with a visual impairment are turning to electronic devices, tablets and smartphones to either complement their current optical aids[1] or to simply replace them altogether. In recent years, there has been a surge in the development of affordable **electronic vision enhancement systems** (EVES) from 'traditional' CCTV desktop systems to tablets and smartphones with accessibility applications offering assistance to people with a visual impairment.

Due to the rapid advancement of technology, any chapter of current products, hardware or applications would go out of date rapidly. Therefore, only the development and generic attributes of EVES are covered here and the low vision practitioner is directed to current suppliers for an up-to-date list of developments.

Electronic vs. optical magnification

Electronic magnification, (real image or transverse magnification) is a method of capturing, enhancing and displaying a magnified image of an object on a display, screen or monitor. It may be calculated by comparing the size of the image on the screen compared to the size of the original object. One of the most significant advantages of using an EVES over an optical device is the ability to manipulate and thus enhance the visibility of the image. The magnification so produced is aberration free, but the quality of the components within the device will determine the quality of the image output, such as the screen resolution.

One of the major disadvantages of using an optical device is that at the higher levels of magnification, patients often find it difficult to keep the image in focus. A steady lens-object distance is required and to improve the field of view, it is also necessary to get in closer to the device. This may be difficult or uncomfortable for many patients to physically achieve.

Most of these characteristics are less relevant when using an electronic device. For example, most desktop or portable EVES are positioned at a fixed distance directly upon or above the object. The field of view is dependent largely upon the size of the screen and not the patient's distance from it. Patients can retain a binocular view and a relatively normal head and body posture whilst viewing the screen. This is an attractive feature for those suffering with a central scotoma or patchy media who find that they need to move their head around to catch an eccentric view of the object.

Reading speed & duration

The success of any device given for sustained reading tasks can be determined in part by the patient's reading speed. Patients report that they are able to read for longer periods of time compared with traditional optical devices.[1,2] The effectivity of different types of electronic devices on reading speed has been studied in clinical trials with mouse EVES connected to a head mounted display resulting in the lowest reading speeds and the more traditional stand EVES with desktop monitor viewing resulting in the best results.[3]

Although EVES can provide benefits in reading speed and acuity some specific tasks can still be performed just as well using optical magnification.[3]

Some of the generic advantages of electronic devices over optical aids are listed below:

- Higher levels of magnification compared to optical devices
- Variable magnification
- Aberration free
- Improved field of view
- Binocular view
- Improved posture: less critical eye-screen working distance
- Manipulation of the image e.g. enhanced contrast options and reverse polarity

History of development

Closed-circuit television systems (CCTVs) were initially developed as surveillance systems used widely since the Second World War. The term 'closed-circuit' describes the direct connection between the camera that captures the image, to the output displayed on a monitor viewing system, rather than an output to a wider audience through broadcast television. The concept behind the use of a CCTV system to create electronic magnification as a method of vision enhancement, was historically first envisaged in the late 1950's.[4,5] However, the high cost of equipment and lack of portability limited its widespread use across the visually impaired population.

As new developments entered the marketplace, the technology behind both the capture and the display of images has continued to evolve. The term electronic vision enhancement systems (EVES) has replaced the term CCTV as a more accurate generic descriptor of the wide variety of devices now in use.[3,6]

A search on the Internet for electronic magnification aids reveals a vast and varied market of products. Devices vary in size, price and degree of complexity, from the larger, traditional desk-mounted apparatus to small, portable devices. The market is expanding rapidly. Some devices not only make use of magnification, but also incorporate methods of digitally capturing, encoding and converting scanned handwritten or printed text documents into electronic files. The data captured may then be converted to synthetic speech or printed in Braille for those who desire additional sensory output.

Classification of EVES

Assistive technology for people with a visual impairment is therefore a rapidly changing marketplace, making classification difficult. Devices are available as electronic mobility aids, night vision aids, obstacle avoidance aids and panning and zooming devices to name but a few. When considering electronic magnification devices however, the following features can be used to describe or classify EVES:

- Methods of image capture (input) and processing
  Camera, digital imaging system, mouse-style camera
- Display (output) device
  Type of screen, monitor, projector, integral display or externally connected
- Methods of display presentation
  Head mounted, stand monitor, portable display
- Incorporated image enhancement features
  Reverse contrast, scrolling text, contrast enhancement
  Audio output, output to Braille printer
  Wi-Fi enabled, multimedia, social media connectivity
- User interface controls
  Voice activation, gesture activation
- Power supply
  Battery type, mains charge

Common features

The list below contains some of the generic features of EVES, which may vary according to the type of monitor and degree of complexity of the device:

- Zoom capability – a range of variable magnification is useful if the VA changes
- Pivotal screens to assist posture
- Full colour, black & white screen
- Self-focusing
- Increased depth of focus with some models enables bulky or curved surfaces to be viewed
- Enhanced contrast, reverse contrast and colour contrast options (e.g. yellow on blue combinations)

- Edge enhancement technology, customised (user-specific) contrast enhancement at different spatial frequencies
- Horizontal or vertical masking
- Highlighting or underlining
- Moveable/ removable reading table
- Split screen view
- Integration with other assistive technology, computer, TV screen, Braille output, audio output
- Freeze-frame facility
- Ability to capture store digital images
- Wi-Fi enabled, multimedia applications
- Automatic or manual scrolling text with variable speed options
- User interface (control) options e.g. voice control, foot pedal controls, gesture activation
- Mains, rechargeable and battery power supplies

Variable magnification

Most electronic devices offer a range of magnification levels, with the largest screens offering the greatest range. This will benefit users who have a wide-ranging number of tasks of different sizes, comparing favourably with the vast majority of optical devices, which tend to offer only a single level of magnification. A range of magnification is also useful if the patient's VA is variable or likely to change.

Screen size and field of view

With optical magnification, the closer the patient can hold the plus lens to the eye, the greater will be the field of view and the greater the number of characters visible for that device. In using a screen to view the magnified image, the field of view is not influenced by the eye-monitor distance, unless the patient is very close, when the reverse becomes true.

Both the field of view and the magnification of the system will be largely dependent upon the screen size. Reducing the screen size will therefore result in a smaller number of characters visible at a given level of magnification.

Contrast, contrast polarity and colour contrast options

Increasing or enhancing the contrast of the text does have an impact upon reading performance. The magnification may then be slightly reduced, improving field of view and reading speeds.[7]

Many patients report that the use of contrast polarity (image reversal) is more visually comfortable when reading. By reversing the text contrast from black on white to white on black, there is a reduction in light scatter within the eye, which has been shown to improve reading performance in a significant number of patients and especially in those who have media opacities or who are photosensitive.[8,9]

Colour contrast options are available with many devices, although at the time of writing there is no evidence to suggest that reading performance may be improved with specific colours.[10] The choice of specific colours by some users may be more down to subjective preferences and individual visual comfort whilst reading.[11]

Practitioners therefore should advise patients to try both the image enhancement and contrast polarity options together when using a device, which may result in less magnification required to perform reading or text-based tasks.

Methods of presenting text

With both optical and electronic magnification, patients report difficulty navigating from the end of one line to the start of the next. Alternative methods of displaying magnified text have been explored that may result in less navigational demand for some patients:

Horizontal scrolling (or drifting) text: requires smooth pursuit and saccadic eye movements.

Rapid serial visual presentation (RSVP): Has been shown to improve reading speeds although the preference is for the patients to have manual control over the speed of word presentation rather than view the text by means of automatic presentation.

Both scrolling text and RSVP have been shown to improve reading speeds although both are less effective when used by patients with central visual loss.[12]

Traditional EVES

Based upon the original CCTV, the principle components of a stand, or desktop EVES with monitor view includes a camera, a light source, a moveable X-Y platform upon which the object is placed, and a monitor or display-screen on which is projected the image. With the larger, wider screen sizes, patients benefit from either an increase in image size and/or an improvement in the field of view (Figure 9.1).

Desktop EVES can be used to view a wide variety of objects including books, magazines, newspapers and colour photographs. If the X-Y platform is removable, patients may be able to place the documents directly onto a desk surface and use the device with a pen for tasks such as form-filling or writing cards, although some have reported spatial difficulties in hand-eye co-ordination, with the need to view a screen whilst using a pen.[12]

This type of unit may also be used for eccentric viewing training; by using appropriately placed markers on the screen, patients are encouraged to eccentrically view object or text. The movable X-Y tables may also be employed in training steady eye strategy, where the object is moved rather than the eye or magnifier (eccentric viewing and steady eye strategy, Chapter 10).

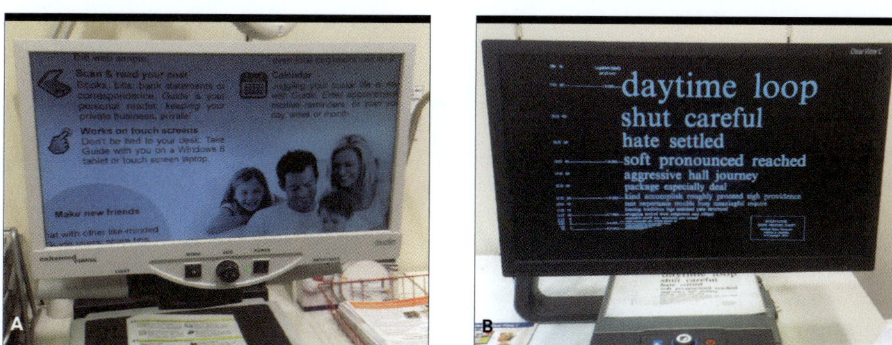

Figure 9.1 Desktop EVES. Reading material is placed upon a moveable X-Y table and projected onto the integrated screen or monitor.
A) The Merlin from *Enhanced Vision.* Coloured text has been captured to produce an enhanced black/white image
B) The ClearView from *Optelec* in reverse contrast mode.

As with most of these traditional devices, the size and weight of the system restricts the user to one place in the home or workplace.

A desktop monitor placed at a habitual and natural viewing distance will assist good posture during use. It also offers binocularity, which is not an option when using high-powered optical aids, as previously mentioned. As a result, prolonged tasks may be more comfortable and manageable, although as with any computer use, patients need to be advised on the importance of taking appropriate breaks. A suitable reading/intermediate addition for the relevant working distance may be appropriate for presbyopic viewers if viewing the screen at a working distance of approximately 1m or less.

Head-mounted devices

The first head mounted device (HMD) was the Low Vision Enhancement System (LVES).[13,14] The original LVES units were heavy but over the years the development of smaller and more efficient components have resulted in a gradual reduction in overall size and weight of units.

The development of HMDs has widened the range of magnification from near to distance objects.[15] A head-mounted unit will allow for a potentially binocular, wide field of view and a 'hands-free' experience for the user. The level of magnification and the number of incorporated image-enhancing features depend upon the complexity of the device. The user interface may consist of a hand-held control unit or may use voice or gesture activation.

HMD's take the form of either spectacle-mounted units or wrap-around goggles with some units permitting the incorporation of refractive error. Where screens are presented immediately in front of the eyes, the increase in magnification will also increase retinal image motion. This can disturb the vestibulo-ocular reflex that would normally limit retinal image instability during head movement. In susceptible individuals, this retinal image 'slip' is known to cause disorientation and symptoms of sea-sickness.[16] In motivated patients this can be overcome by a period of training and adaptation.[17]

There are a number of different methods of HMD screen technologies incorporated into devices. Virtual reality (VR) displays, also known as immersive displays, have been traditionally used in the entertainment industry; users are immersed in a 3-dimensional simulated world. See-through displays, or augmented reality (AR), superimpose images onto the user's field of view, either via a see-through display just in front of the eye or by directly projecting the image onto the retina. The AR method allows the patient to experience habitual vision whilst benefiting from the additional information on the display.[18]

Customisable image enhancement is also now possible. For example, it is possible to target and thus enhance specific spatial frequencies relating to specific visual tasks such as face recognition.[19]

For near tasks, however, HMDs have been less successful, with most of the development now focused upon intermediate and distance tasks. A reduction in reading speed and performance of near tasks is demonstrably seen using HMDs compared with desktop style EVES.[3]

Development of portable systems

Over recent years, more portable magnifiers have become available, offering good quality images at a lower cost than desktop systems. Unfortunately, a number of companies have developed and produced devices without the appropriate research and development that is required to create a device specifically for people with a visual impairment, many of whom have reduced manual dexterity and/or reduced cognitive ability.[20]

Portable EVES, or p-EVES,[20] offer electronic vision enhancement with many of the accompanying benefits without the restraints of the space and weight of larger desk-top systems. Portable systems are targeted for day-to-day tasks with the flexibility to be used in different locations. For both short tasks, such as checking medication, to more sustained near tasks, such as reading the newspaper, devices provide a relatively inexpensive, cosmetically acceptable low vision aid with many of the image enhancement features available in the larger, less portable devices (Figure 9.2).

Designs and functionality vary across manufacturers and include hand-held portable units with integral screens or those that include the use of an optical mouse connected to a monitor or separate screen such as a television.

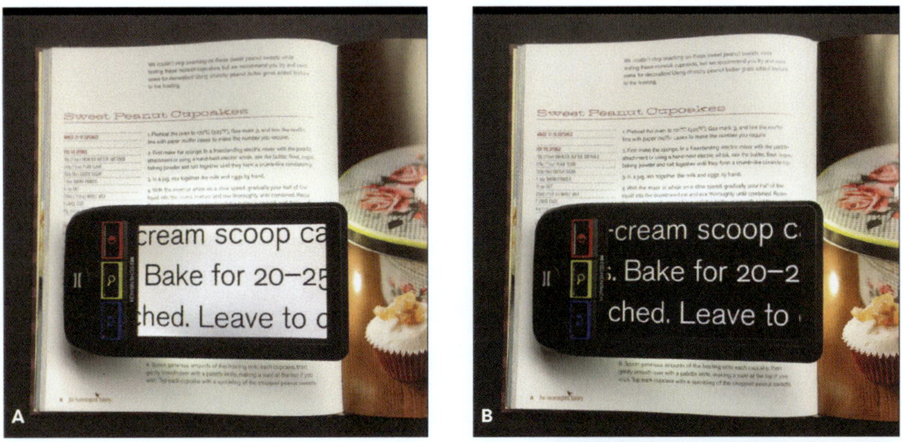

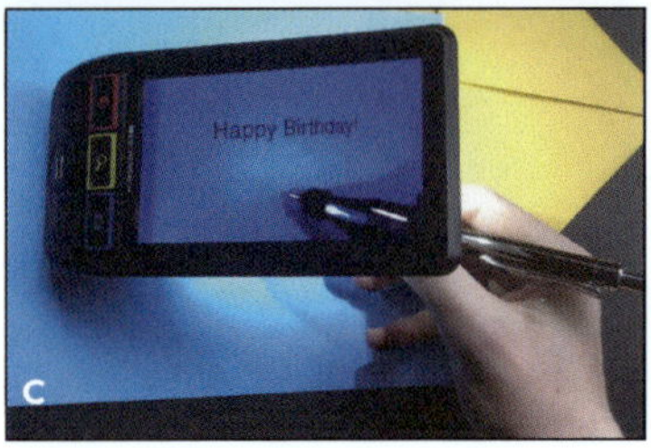

Figure 9.2 *Eschenbach's* portable Smartlux Digital **A)** the wider screen offers the viewer potentially more words or letters horizontally. **B)** Reverse contrast mode. **C)** The integral stand may be adjusted to allow the use of a pen.

p-EVES and spectacle correction

When using portable devices, most patients will opt to use their device at a their previous 'habitual' reading distance. Therefore, they may benefit from using their reading correction. It is not unusual to see some patients use a higher reading addition or spectacle lens magnifier in combination with an electronic device. In this instance, the resultant magnification will be a product of both the spectacle magnifier and the magnification produced on the screen.

Software & applications

Tablets, smartphone devices, eBook readers and computers offer people with a visual impairment accessibility features such as large print, image enhancement, reverse contrast and speech output.

Third-party applications and specialist computer software offer magnification options; GPS led navigation applications assist with independent travel, and audiobook or eBooks offer the user alternative methods of listening or reading novels or magazines. Voice activated and controlled methods of sending and listening to text improves communication and enables browsing the Internet.

Summary

The advancements and improvements in the quality and efficiency of components have widened the use of electronic magnification. All age groups are now regular computer users and as relative costs reduce and portability improves many predict that domestic use will become commonplace. Rigorous testing of new and emerging technologies is vital, alongside discussion with end-user groups on the functionality of a new device. Systematic, high-quality research is also necessary to assess the effectiveness of new technologies and compare them with existing methods already in use. All too often new products appear in the marketplace, with the promise of something 'different' for people with a visual impairment. However, few of these devices undergo the rigorous research that is required to determine whether or not it will be a successful rehabilitative device for a person with reduced vision. Just as important is the requirement of acceptability of the device in terms of appearance, comfort and ease of use.[15]

The long-term success of any new device within the marketplace is not only determined by improved visual function such as acuity, reading speed or contrast sensitivity, but also whether or not the device enables the user to perform a range of daily living activities and thus improve their overall quality of life.

The number of EVES, p-EVES and HMDs in the marketplace is slowly increasing. In time, older patients may turn to electronic magnification as a fundamental

method of magnification, but whether it replaces optical magnification altogether is questionable. However, low vision practitioners should be able to discuss the advantages of electronic devices and other complimentary devices such as smartphones and tablets alongside the established optical approach to prescribing magnification during the consultation and where appropriate, refer onto services that are able to address the patient's needs in this area.

References

1. Goodrich GL, Mehr EB, Darling NC. Parameters in use of CCTV and optical Aids. Am J Optom Physiol Opt. 1980;57:881–92.
2. Uslan M, Shen R, Shragai Y. The evolution of video magnification technology. J Vis Impair Blind. 1996;90:465–78.
3. Peterson RC, Wolffsohn JS, Rubinstein M, Lowe J. Benefits of electronic vision enhancement systems (EVES) for the visually impaired. Am J Ophthalmol. 2003;136(6):1129–35.
4. Potts AM, Volk D, West SS. A television reader as a subnormal vision aid. Am J Ophthalmol. 1959;47:580–1.
5. Genensky SM, Baran P, Moshin HL, Steingold H. A closed circuit TV system for the visually handicapped. RAND Corp. 1968;
6. Wolffsohn JS, Peterson RC. A review of current knowledge on Electronic Vision Enhancement Systems for the visually impaired. Ophthalmic Physiol Opt. 2003;23(1):35–42.
7. Brown B. Reading performance in low vision patients: relation to contrast and contrast sensitivity. Optom Vis Sci. 1981;
8. Legge GE, Rubin GS, Schleske MM. Contrast polarity effects in low vision reading. In: Low Vision. New York, NY: Springer New York; 1987. p. 288–307.
9. Rubin G, Legge G. Psychophysics of reading-VI The role of contrast in low vision. Vision Res. 1989;29(1):79–91.
10. Legge GE, Rubin GS. Psychophysics of reading-IV Wavelength effects in normal and low vision. J Opt Soc Am A. 1986;3(1):40–51.
11. Jacobs RJ. Screen color and reading performance on closed-circuit television. J Vis Impair Blind. 1990;84(10):569–72.

12. Harland S, Legge GE, Luebker A. Psychophysics of reading-XVII Low-vision performance with four types of electronically magnified text. Optom Vis Sci. 1998;75(3).

13. Massof R, Rickman D. Obstacles encountered in the development of the low vision enhancement system. Optom Vis Sci. 1992;69(31–41).

14. Massof RW, Rickman DL, Lalle PA. Low vision enhancement system. Johns Hopkins APL Tech Dig (Applied Phys Lab. 1994;15(2):120–5.

15. Harper R, Culham L, Dickinson C. Head mounted video magnification devices for low vision rehabilitation: a comparison with existing technology. Br J Ophthalmol. 1999;83(4):495–500.

16. Peli E. The visual effects of head mounted display HMD are not distinguishable from those desk top computer display. Vision Res. 1998;38:2053–66.

17. Demer JL, Porter FI, Goldberg J, Jenkins HA, Schmidt K. Dynamic visual acuity with telescopic spectacles: Improvement with adaptation. Investig Ophthalmol Vis Sci. 1988;29(7):1184–9.

18. Ehrlich JR, Ojeda L V, Wicker D, Day S, Howson A, Lakshminarayanan V, et al. Head-mounted display technology for low vision rehabilitation and vision enhancement. Am J Ophthalmol. 2017;26–32.

19. Peli E, Goldstein R, Young G. Image enhancement for the visually impaired. Invest Ophthalmol Vis Sci. 1991;32:2337–50.

20. Taylor J, Bambrick R, Dutton M, Harper R, Ryan B, Tudor-Edwards R, et al. The p-EVES study design and methodology: a randomised controlled trial to compare portable electronic vision enhancement systems (p-EVES) to optical magnifiers for near vision activities in visual impairment. Ophthalmic Physiol Opt. 2014;34(34):558–72.

CHAPTER TEN

Additional Strategies, Non-optical Aids and Lighting

> "Lighting of objects and rooms is important and often overlooked. For people with poor visual acuity and poor contrast sensitivity, optimal lighting is often the only variable that can be improved easily."
>
> **David Elks BSc MCOptom**

Additional Strategies, Non-optical Aids and Lighting

Introduction

Alongside the prescribing of an optical magnification device such as a hand magnifier or a telescope, there are a number of additional approaches or strategies, aids to daily living or adaptations to the environment that assist people with a visual impairment to maintain independence following sight loss. This chapter outlines alternative methods used to enhance visual performance and describes some of the additional strategies used for specific pathological conditions that acquire further assistance or a unique approach.

Big, Bright and Bold: methods of improving object visibility

- **Big:** increasing the size of objects using various or combined methods of magnification
- **Bright:** increasing the visibility of the object by the use of additional lighting
- **Bold:** improving the visibility of the object using colour and contrast

Relative size magnification

The retinal image is increased by enlarging the physical size of the object. A comparison can be made between the new object size and old object size to determine the overall magnification effect:

$$\text{Magnification} = \frac{\text{New object size}}{\text{Old object size}}$$

Increasing the physical size of an object or text is possible for many items, however, this is only realistic for low levels of magnification; for example, producing a television screen to be twice its original size is both expensive and often impractical. Similarly, household items, games or books, etc. may all be produced larger, but with a practical limitation of approximately 1½-2½ x original size.

Large print

Most printed reading material for adult use is produced in approximately N8–N12 over a wide variety of font styles. Large print books and newspapers are typically N18–N24, which is roughly 2x larger than standard print. When producing large print materials, the choice of typeface, level of contrast and the colours used in printing are equally important as factors that improve the overall legibility of the text. However, these factors often add to the total cost of publication.

Large print books are an option with older patients; normal reading posture and binocularity may be maintained, and for those only requiring low levels of magnification, they may still be able to read with the book on their lap. No special training or advice is necessary when this method is chosen. Many patients may also combine methods of magnification to assist reading. For example, using a hand magnifier whilst reading a large print newspaper.

Combining magnifications

Where more than one method of magnification is used in combination, e.g. using a 3x hand magnifier in combination with 2x enlarged print, the overall magnification is a product of the two, which in this example would be the equivalent of 6x.

To produce 2½ x magnification in large print, the book or newspaper itself will physically increase in size. Publications produced in large print are therefore heavier and bulkier. The use of thinner paper can be used, but if the paper used is too thin, the print from the underlying pages becomes visible and hence either bothersome or impossible to use. Abridged versions of novels will reduce the overall size of the book but are, by rights of publication, often unacceptable. Children may benefit from enlarging schoolwork or printed text larger. Public examination papers are often made available to students in alternative formats including large print. Care must be taken when successive photocopying is used to produce enlargement as this may cause a reduction in the quality and contrast of the material. The best practice is to transcribe into large print rather than to photocopy.

Examples of relative size magnification

- Large print books, novels, textbooks, reference books, sheet music
- Maps, catalogues, bus timetables,
- Diaries, calendars, telephone book
- Puzzle books, crosswords, Sudoku
- Board games, e.g. Scrabble, Monopoly, dominoes and jumbo playing cards
- Bank statements, utility bills
- Large print and auditory greeting cards
- Large face clocks and watches
- Large button telephones, large button keyboards
- Large button mobile phones

Colour contrast

Colour contrast can be used as a practical approach to various recognition tasks.[1,2] It improves the speed and accuracy of naming familiar objects and can be indispensable to many who live alone, improving safety and lessening the degree of frustration.

Examples of colour-contrast

- A coloured bar of soap against a white sink
- Serving tea or coffee in a white mug
- Serving white fish on a dark coloured plate

Colour discrimination is often affected by acquired visual impairment. For example, colours may appear washed out or faded. The use of brightly coloured markers can assist in the identification of everyday household objects or items. High-visibility, tactile markers or bands, produced in a variety of bright colours and sizes, may be used to highlight anything such as cooker dials, switches, tins and bottles (Figure 10.1). Coloured buttons of various shapes may be sewn into clothing to aid identification. Brightly coloured tape may be used to demarcate the edges of internal obstacles, such as steps or the edges of tables.

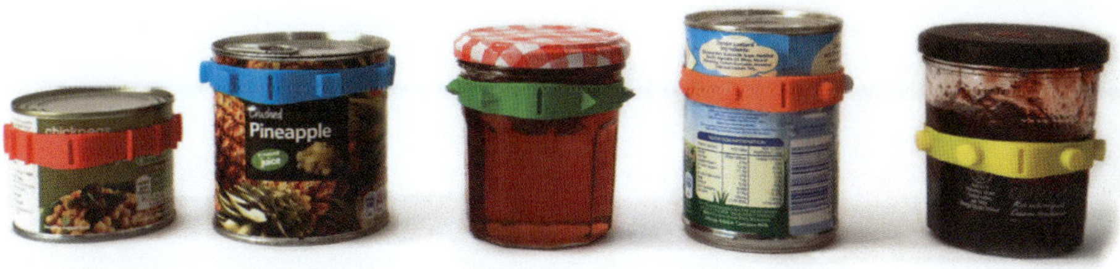

Figure 10.1 Bright coloured bands with raised tactile shapes may be used around the home to mark specific items such as food tins or medication. Image courtesy of Hannah Scoones, *Band-it*

Contrast polarity

Increasing or enhancing the contrast of text has been shown to improve reading performance. The magnification may then be slightly reduced, improving the field of view and reading speeds.[3] Many patients report that the use of contrast polarity printed text (white text on a black background) is more visually comfortable when reading. This may be produced digitally, for example, using Electronic Vision Enhancement Systems (EVES, Chapter 9). By reversing the text polarity, the resultant reduction in light scatter within the eye has been shown to improve reading performance in a significant number of patients and especially in those who have media opacities or those who are photosensitive.[4,5]

The Prentice Typoscope

Charles Prentice first described his 'typo-scope' in 1897. The simplicity of using a piece of black card with a cut-out slit has the effect of reducing the scatter of excess light in a similar way to using the reverse polarity function on an EVES. Depending on the size of the hole or slit, which is cut into the black card or sheet, one or several lines of print may be 'highlighted'. The typoscope additionally aids tracking and is often used with eccentric viewing or steady eye strategy techniques. Patients who successfully use a typoscope often demonstrate improvement in reading performance (Figure 10.2).

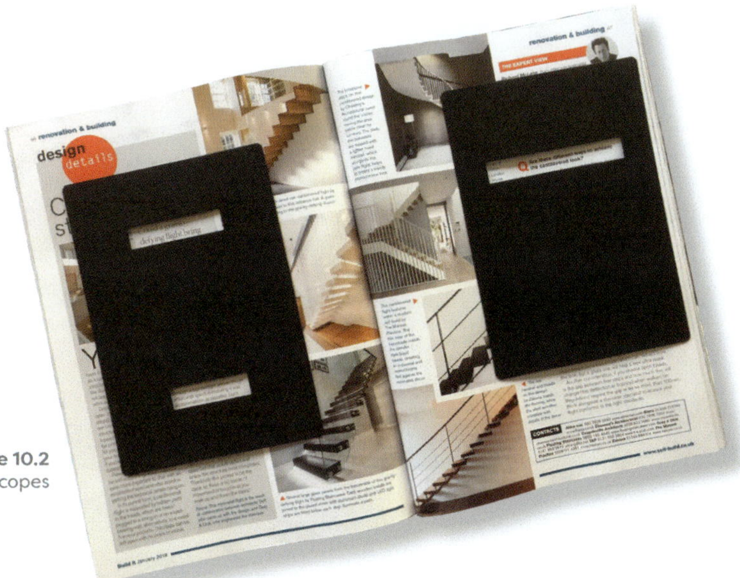

Figure 10.2
Prentice typoscopes

Auditory and tactile: using other senses

A large number of the non-optical aids discussed or listed in this chapter incorporate the use of additional 'stimuli' such as touch or sound to enhance the functionality of the aid. For example talking kitchen scales, clocks, vibrating watches and raised tactile markers or bands (Figure 10.1).

- Auditory – e.g. beeps, bells, whistles, voice
- Tactile – e.g. embossed or raised surfaces, vibration

Aids for daily living

The ability to continue with day-to-day living tasks is fundamental to independence and quality of life. Activities of daily living such as meal preparation, cooking and personal hygiene become significant challenges following even a mild loss of vision. Safety is of paramount importance from slicing bread or peeling vegetables to pouring hot liquids or checking whether meat is thoroughly cooked or not. Such tasks most of us take for granted, but understanding whether or not a loaf of bread is mouldy is not a simple task when the vision is poor. Rehabilitation teams offer practical advice in and around the home and will 'markup' appliances such as the cooker, washing machine or microwave with raised, high contrast, tactile coloured markers (occasionally known as 'bump-ons') to assist programme choice or to simply understand whether or not the appliance has been safely turned off.

There are a large number of aids to daily living for people with a visual impairment. Some aids may be issued by rehabilitation teams or are available to buy from resource centres. Successful products have been carefully designed and developed in association with patient focus groups, such as the award-winning debit card seen in Figure 10.3. A list of some of the popular items for everyday living and personal care, many of which incorporate the use of other senses, is included below:

- Audible and vibratory liquid level indicators
- Talking scales, measuring jugs, food thermometers and kitchen timers
- One-touch tin openers, talking tin lids
- Writing guides, signature guides, chequebook covers,
- Thick pens and markers, thick-lined stationery
- Bread cutter boards and safety peelers
- Talking calculators
- Large button TV remote with voice activation or output
- Self-adhesive tactile markers and bands for the cooker, washing machine, sockets and household items
- Coin and banknote holders
- Talking microwave
- Pill dispensers
- Voice labelling recorders, memo recorders
- Large and high contrast keyboards
- Magnifying mirrors
- Eye drop dispensers
- Talking blood glucose and blood pressure monitors
- High visibility tape and edge markers

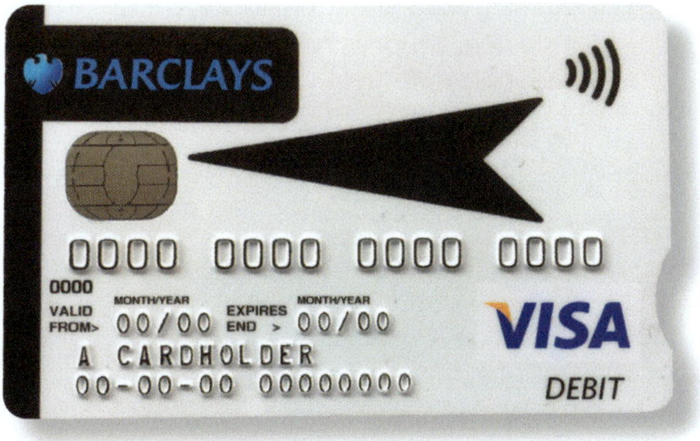

Figure 10.3
A debit card designed for people with a visual impairment. A notch at the base of the card assists users with inserting the card into payment machines and cash dispensers in the correct direction. Cards are available in high contrast and bold colours. With thanks to Louise Pearson, Barclays UK

Talking books and newspapers

Most libraries and organisations supporting people with a visual impairment, have either produced or have access to a broad range of talking books, talking newspapers and accessible learning resources. These are produced in a variety of audio formats and for a range of devices including smartphones and electronic book readers.

Tactile codes: Braille

Braille has been in use since it was first devised by Louis Braille in 1824. It was based upon a tactile military code using sets of embossed dots. The code is based on six dots, arranged in two columns of three dots, with 63 possible combinations.

The majority of Braille readers have been taught Braille from an early age. For those with an acquired visual impairment in later life, learning the technique can be slow and difficult, especially if the fingertips have become less sensitive over time. The number of Braille readers has gradually decreased in recent years due to an increase in alternative methods of assistive technology. Therefore the number of regular Braille readers is small, with estimates ranging from 1-10% of the visual impairment population regularly using the technique. Books are bulky, and there is a limited choice of titles. It is estimated that only 7% of books are available in large print, audio and Braille formats combined.[6]

Management of photophobia and glare: tints & filters

Photophobia and glare sensitivity are commonly encountered in patients with a visual impairment. Exposure to different types of light and lighting can be uncomfortable, painful or may cause a further reduction in visual acuity. This will have functional implications for a number of patients. Examples of some conditions or circumstances that may give rise to chronic photophobia or long-term glare sensitivity include:[7]

- Corneal pathologies, including dystrophies, abrasion or trauma
- Corneal scarring following surgical intervention
- Posterior segment disease, e.g. uveitis
- Anterior segment disease, e.g. iritis,
- Cataract and other media opacities
- Albinism
- Diabetic retinopathy
- Macular degeneration
- Macular dystrophy
- Rod and cone dystrophies, e.g. retinitis pigmentosa, achromatopsia
- Glaucoma
- CNS disorders such as meningitis, progressive supranuclear palsy (PSP)
- Brain injuries, lesions,
- Migraine

Note: The term photophobia is often used widely by practitioners to describe any sensitivity to light. Strictly speaking, true photophobia is caused by an underlying pathology resulting in symptoms such as pain or extreme discomfort, tearing and blepharospasm.[7]

Many people experience an increased sensitivity to glare as they age due to an increase in media opacities. Glare can be caused by sunlight, other lighting sources, or reflections. There are two definitions of glare: discomfort glare and disability glare.

With **discomfort glare**, the patient complains that the light within his or her visual field is excessively bright and is causing discomfort. There will be a higher level of luminance entering the eye to that currently adapted, and the discomfort may impede functional performance.

The effect of **disability glare** is to impair the patient's visual performance. For example, a cataract may cause a scatter of light when there is high ambient illumination, and the eye will experience a drop in acuity.

In addition, **reflection glare** from a smooth surface can occur to people with both normal and impaired vision when reading a shiny page of a book or magazine. When the angle of incident light is equal to the angle of reflected light entering the eye, the surface acts like a mirror, and the print becomes obscured. This is known as specular reflection and will occur on all smooth or polished surfaces (the term specular is derived from the Latin word speculum, meaning 'mirror'). A shift in the position of either the book or the reader will change the angle of either the incident beam or reflected light, and the masking of the print is removed (Figure 10.4).

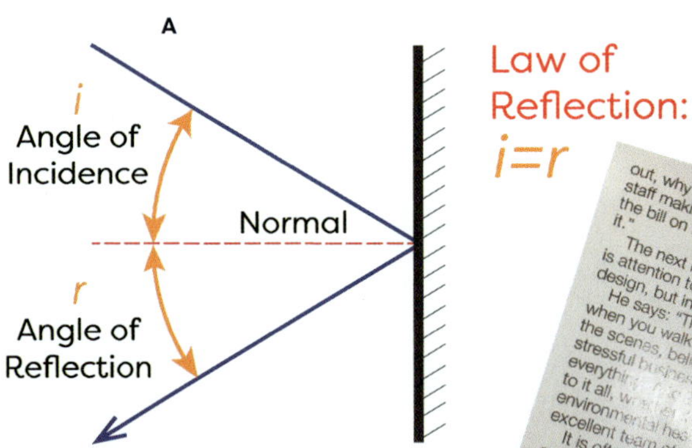

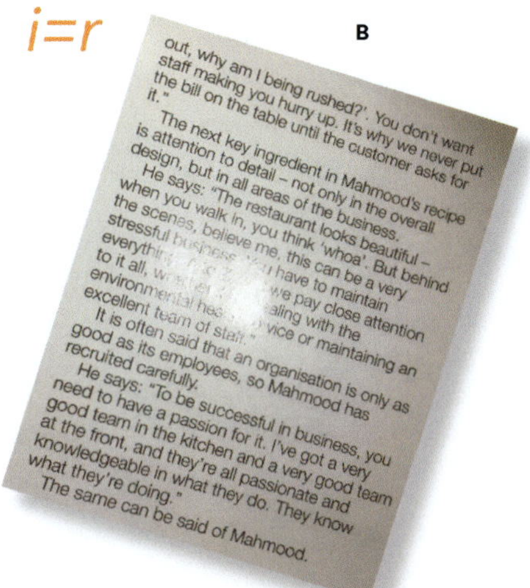

Figure 10.4 A Specular reflection
A) the angle of incident light (i), equals the angle of reflected light (r), resulting in specular reflection from a smooth surface. If the surface was not smooth the reflected light would become scattered and diffuse
B) the patch of specularly reflected light from the page of a glossy magazine obscures the text beneath

Management of glare

Ideally, the management of photophobia or glare sensitivity will focus on removing or reducing the underlying cause. For example:

- Treatment or removal of the underlying pathological cause
- Elimination or reduction of the light source or the scattered light
- Change of position
- Obstructing the light source using visors, shields, hats and caps

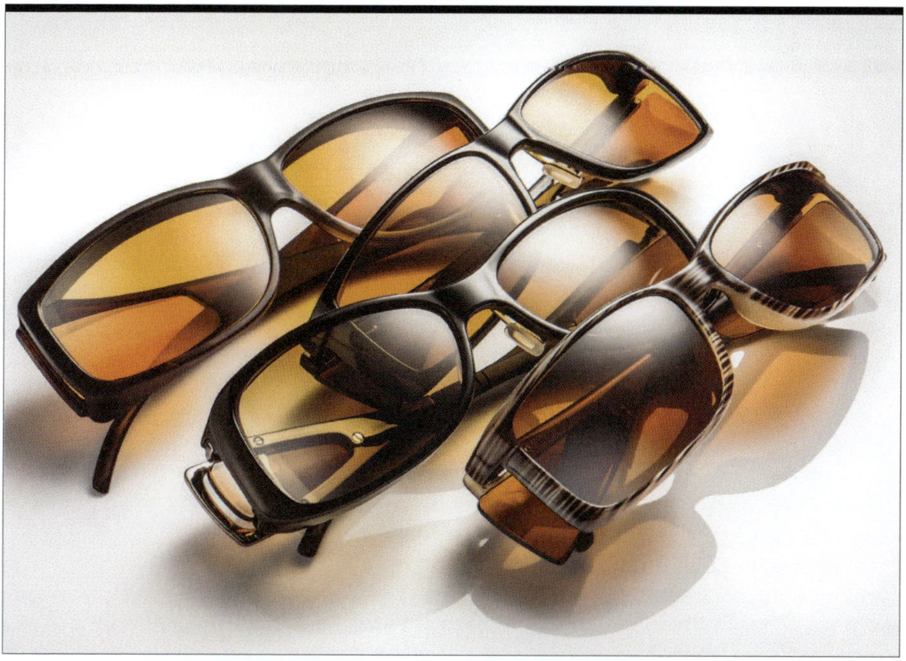

Figure 10.5 wellnessPROTECT® range of glasses from *Eschenbach* may be additionally glazed to the patient's prescription or used as over-spectacles. Brow-line and side shielding offer additional glare protection. Lenses offer absorption of UV and short wavelength light.

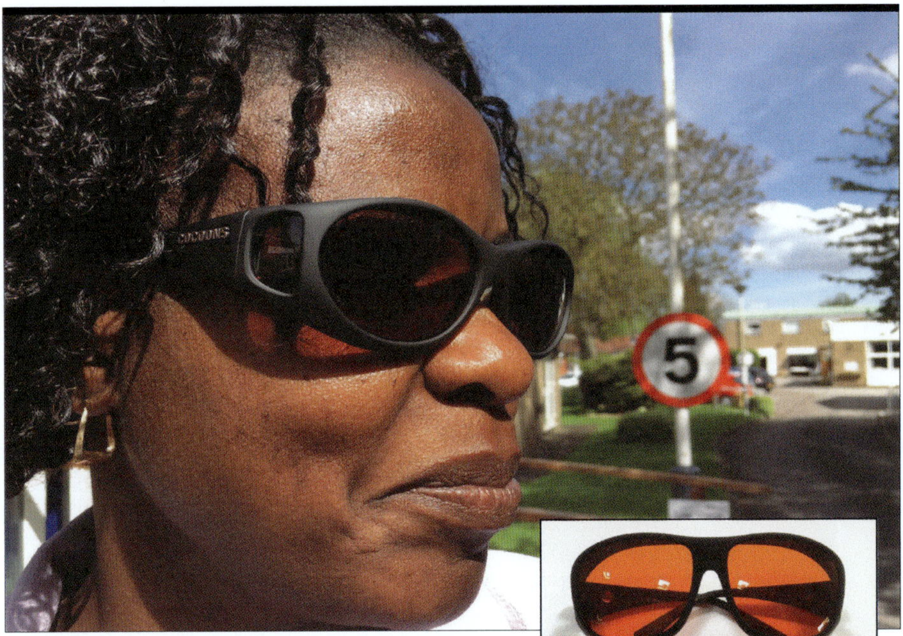

Figure 10.6 Filtered over-spectacles from *Cocoon*

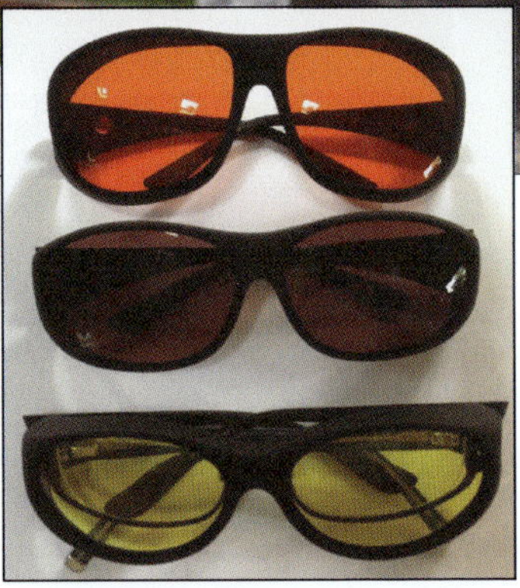

Over-spectacles and filters

Any tint may be useful in bright sunlight, just as sunglasses are useful on a sunny day, by reducing the amount of light entering the eye (Figures 10.5 & 10.6). However, a dark tint may impair visual function indoors or when levels of illumination are low which can become hazardous for people with a visual impairment. Wrap-around sunglasses have the additional advantage of reducing unwanted sources from the sides. Photochromic lenses are often suggested as one of the better solutions to reduce the undesirable effects of discomfort glare. However, the usefulness of these lenses will be dependent on how effective their reactions are in both bright sunlight and dim indoor illumination. Polarised lenses may reduce specular reflection from surfaces such as water, allowing a fisherman to see fish beneath the surface, but have little effect on overall glare from the sun. Furthermore, the use of polarised lenses impedes the ability to view LCD screens such as those on a smartphone. When discussing tints for discomfort glare, it often comes down to subjective choice by the user and the eyecare practitioner should warn the patient of the limitations of any type used.

Tints to improve visual performance

The primary objective when prescribing a tint for disability glare is to enhance visual performance by selectively absorbing the scattered light and improving retinal image contrast. This is difficult to achieve with a tint, as this necessitates selective absorption characteristics of the tint. The evidence on the use of tinted lenses and filters for improving visual performance, such as reading speed, acuity or contrast sensitivity, raises mixed results and is often ambiguous. So it is not surprising that feedback from patients gives very mixed results.[8] Despite this, several manufacturers and low vision suppliers offer an extensive range of coloured tints and filters that claim improvement in performance, often with reference to specific pathological conditions despite having little or no supporting scientific evidence.

In contrast, however, low vision practitioners frequently come across individuals who report marked subjective preferences whilst using specific filters to improve visual comfort whilst reading or whilst mobile out of doors. Practitioners should, therefore, remain sensitive to patient's individual preferences and at least be able to offer a balanced view of the current claims.

Lighting for low vision

General lighting

With age, the amount of light entering the eye is reduced. Weale suggested that retinal illumination at the age of 60 is about one third that found at the age of 20.[9] This can have the effect of reducing acuity, contrast perception and colour discrimination.

A large proportion of homes occupied by older people have illumination levels markedly below recommended levels.[10,11] In the majority of cases, the inadequate levels of illumination will result in reduced visual performance for many daily living tasks. Most people with a visual impairment, therefore, benefit from a review of their current lighting solutions, either within the home, work or school environment. Task lighting and general ambient lighting should ideally be optimised to improve both safety and visual performance. This includes a review of the amount, direction and the appropriate shielding of the light and light sources.[12,13] Lighting solutions within the home include low-level lighting on stairs to provide differentiation between treads and risers; correct use of lighting will also improve activities of daily living which in turn has been shown to improve patient's quality of life.[10,14]

Recommended light levels

Standards for lighting levels for public spaces, highways, schools, offices and homes will vary according to the country of origin and is beyond the scope of this text. However, the list below is a guide of various recommended lighting levels for a number of familiar locations or activities:[12,15,16]

Location or activity	Light level
Public areas	20-100 Lux
Working areas where visual tasks are occasionally performed	100-150 Lux
Warehouses, homes, theatres, public toilets	150-300 Lux
Offices and classrooms	250-500 Lux
Optometry consulting rooms	300-500 Lux
PC Work, study, library, showrooms, laboratories	500 Lux
Supermarkets	500-750 Lux
Mechanical workshops, operating theatres	750-1,000 Lux
Detailed intricate or mechanical work	1,500-2,000 Lux
Low contrast visual tasks and small size for prolonged periods	2,000-5,000 Lux
Performance of prolonged and exacting visual tasks	5,000-10,000 Lux
Performance of visual tasks of low contrast and small size	10,000-20,000 Lux

Illuminance levels of approximately 300-500 lux are suggested for sustained reading or sewing for younger patients. This would need to be increased to between 450 lux and 600 lux in older patients over the age of 65 and to 1000 lux or more in patients suffering from a visual impairment such as age-related macular degeneration.[15,17]

Task lighting

Increasing task illuminance has a significant effect on the visual function of both normal and low vision patients,[17–19] but those with a visual impairment require greater illuminance to reach maximum visual performance.[20–22]

Task lighting refers to a localised light source directed onto a specific activity or task. For example in the kitchen, a patient may require under cabinet down lighting for cutting and preparing food. The ratio of the task illuminance to that surrounding should not exceed 3:1. Therefore, significant differences in light levels should be avoided both between the task and the rest of the background. Patients should be recommended to increase room lighting when they increase task lighting and to avoid using a bright lamp in a very dark room.[17]

The Inverse Square Law

The inverse square law describes the intensity of light at different distances from a light source. The intensity of light is inversely proportional to the square of the distance. The same applies to the whole electromagnetic spectrum (visible light, radio waves, microwaves, ultraviolet and infrared, etc.). The intensity of visible light is measured in *candela* units (cd):

Light intensity is proportional to 1/distance squared

$$I \propto 1/d^2$$

Example:
A light source placed at 100cm from a page or object will appear four times as bright when it is moved closer to 50cm.

Using other senses

Aids for orientation and mobility

For those who experience a loss of sight in later life, the loss of independent means of travel out of doors can be devastating.[23] Now unable to drive, people may need to consider the use of public transport, taxis, as well as support from family and friends to assist with getting from one place to the next, such as the weekly grocery shop or hospital appointments. Many individuals may find using an unfamiliar public transport system challenging and often overwhelming.

White sticks and canes

The 'white stick' is universal across the world as a symbol of visual impairment. James Biggs of Bristol, England lost his sight due to an accident, and in 1921 he painted a stick white to make him more visible to the increasing numbers of motorists on the roads. Over the years a number of canes have been developed to assist those with a visual impairment. These are further described in Chapter 12.

Trailing techniques

Trailing techniques are taught to assist patients to move about both indoors and out of doors safely. Patients are trained to use the back of the hand, with fingers slightly cupped towards the palm. Patients use the techniques to 'feel' their way along a wall, or move safely up and down stairs and through doorways.

Other strategies to improve performance

Eccentric viewing and steady eye strategy

The concept of eccentric viewing (EV) training has been in use for some time as a rehabilitative strategy where the patient is trained to use paracentral areas of the retina to fixate an object.[24,25] The majority of patients with central vision loss develop one or more preferred retinal loci (PRL) within six months of vision loss.[26] However, this PRL may not be stable; nor may it be one that can be used to maximise visual ability.[27,28] Therefore some patients may benefit from additional training to select a retinal locus to maximise visual capability, known as the trained retinal locus (TRL)[29] (Figure 10.7).

Figure 10.7 The concept of using an Amsler Grid to eccentrically view an object. The patient is asked to concentrate on the centre of the grid. If the clearest area of the grid is left of centre (9 o'clock) then the patient is asked to look in the opposite direction i.e. right of centre (3 o'clock) so that the clearest area moves into the centre of the grid.

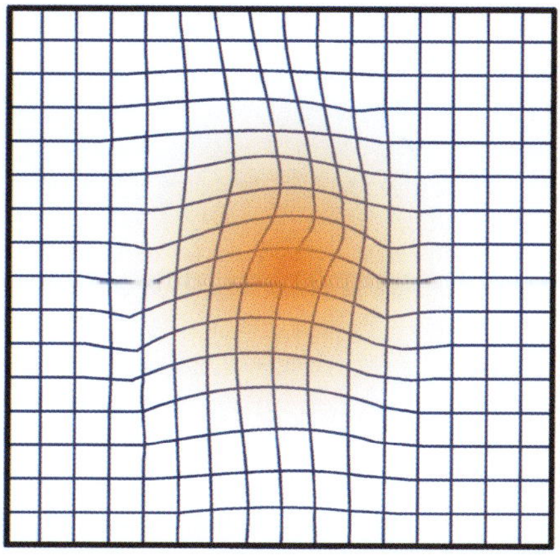

With a reduction in fixation stability following central vision loss,[27,30] the use of steady eye strategy technique (SES) removes the need for saccadic eye movements. The PRL/TRL is directed towards an area of text or a single word and the eye is held in a steady position whilst the text is moved through the fixation point.[31]

Despite a large number of rehabilitation services offering EV and SES training,[32] there is still a lack of evidence regarding effectiveness, with only moderate evidence to suggest that combined EV and SES training improves reading speed and activities of daily living in patients with central vision loss.[29]

Using prism spectacles

The use of using prisms to relocate the retinal image has been shown to have mixed results.[33,34] Prisms are incorporated into the patient's spectacles to relocate the image to the PRL. Some patients report a significant subjective improvement although clinically the improvement in clinical measures such as visual acuity, contrast sensitivity and reading speeds have only been slight.[35]

Enhancement of the visual field

Retinitis Pigmentosa

For those patients with severely restricted visual fields but who retain relatively good central visual acuity, the use of devices that 'expand' the visual field through minification of the visual field has been studied extensively.[36-38] However, few patients make use of the variety of field-expanding devices such as reversed telescopes or high minus lenses[39] (Figure 10.8).

Reports from patients suggest one of two reasons. Functional adaptation to peripheral field loss through the development of scanning techniques can be so efficient, that patients are often unaware of even an extensive loss of visual field for many years. Whilst a patient may have a static 10^{0} visual field measured through traditional visual field examination, scanning techniques may improve this to a dynamic visual field of 50^{0} or more. Secondly, most patients with a severe restriction in their visual field, despite good central acuity, are more concerned about bumping into objects or missing kerbs and steps that are in close proximity. The use of field expanders minify the visual field beyond arm's length and is less likely to highlight obstacles affecting mobility that are close by.

There are times that the field expander is used to significant effect. Examples include watching children

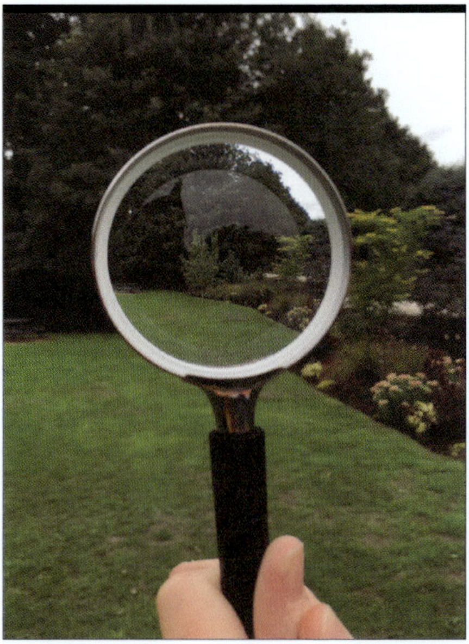

Figure 10.8 Minification of the visual field using a high minus field expander, courtesy of Andy Cook, Sight for Surrey.

in the park or playing a game of rounders or allowing an overview of a football ground. Whilst these examples do not assist the patient in general mobility, the gross overview or general orientation to 'set the scene' is welcomed by several patients. Particularly when in an unfamiliar environment.[40,41] However, it must be remembered that minification is less likely to be used when patients have a drop in central visual acuity.

Hemianopic defects

Hemianopic defects can have a significant impact upon both mobility and reading performance and often represent a considerable challenge to both practitioner and patient. In comparison with patients with a progressive field loss such as that found in retinitis pigmentosa, patients with a hemianopic defect have lost their visual field suddenly and therefore have had less time to adapt.

Defects on the right side of the visual field impact on reading from left to right. Defects on the left side of the visual field can cause problems in locating the start of the next line. Orientation and mobility and activities of daily living can be severely affected, and patients may benefit from training in scanning techniques and compensatory eye movements.[42]

Boundary marking describes a simple method of marking either the end or the beginning of a line with a piece of coloured card whilst reading. For example, a patient with a left homonymous hemianopia should place the coloured card at the start of the line when reading. Patients are encouraged to follow the same line of text back until they reach the boundary marker and then drop down to the next line.

Peripheral prism glasses

Peripheral prism glasses may provide benefit in mobility such as obstacle avoidance for patients with homonymous hemianopia.[43-45] To extend the horizontal visual field, spectacles can be fitted with prism segments across the lens on the side of the visual field loss. There are a number of patented lens styles now available such as the Peli Expansion Prism (Figure 10.9), the Chadwick and the Gottlieb lens.

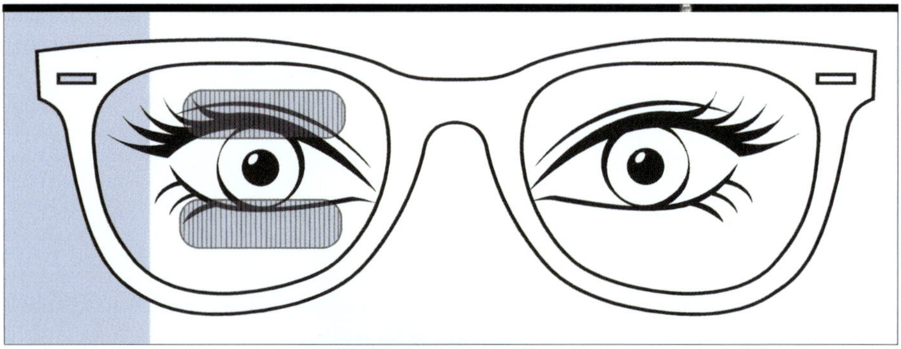

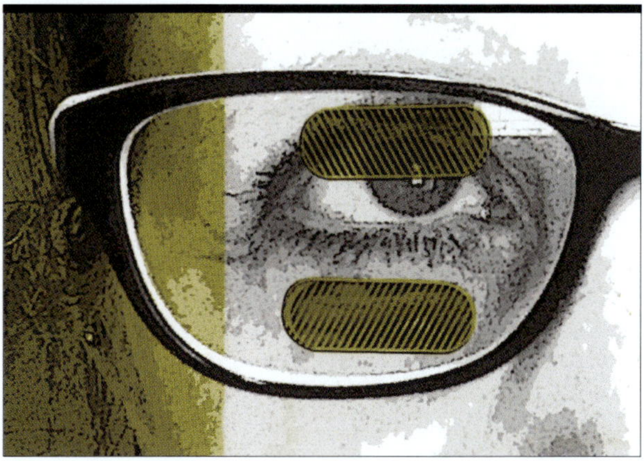

Figure 10.9 The Peli Expansion Prism (EP) Lens.
Above: 40Δ Fresnel prisms are fitted on the side of the visual field loss above and below the optical centre.
Right: The patient is looking up to view the area of visual field loss (shaded) within the prism.

Visual neglect

Hemispatial inattention, or visual neglect, is often confused with homonymous hemianopia although it may occur in association with it. It is not a true visual field defect, and it is better described as a disorder that prevents the patient from attending to stimuli on one side of the body. It can be a consequence of stroke and is considered the result of damage to the posterior parietal lobe of the brain although some authorities argue that the lesion may be mid-brain in origin.[46] A patient with hemispatial inattention, for example, may not respond to a voice when the person is on the left or a man may only shave one side of his face.

Occlusion

Patients regularly report 'interference' from a fellow eye, particularly when the vision in the fellow eye is considerably worse, has extensive distortion or monocular diplopic images. This interference becomes more problematic when trying to use their low vision device or when concentrating on specific tasks such as watching the television. Although some practitioners may suggest the use of a tissue placed behind the lens, this may not be practical especially if the patient is watching the television for extended periods. In these circumstances, much of the interference can be relieved by using an adult orthoptic eye patch which may be simply removed when not in use (Figure 10.10). In cases where the interference is severe, patients may benefit from a more permanent solution such as an occlusive lens in the fellow eye.

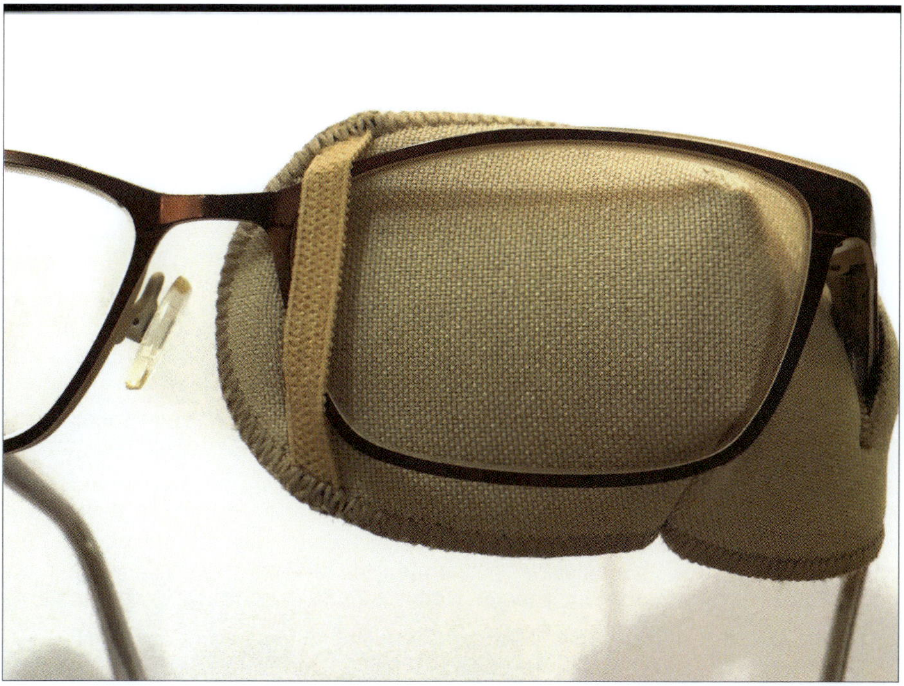

Figure 10.10 An adult orthoptic patch it fitted to the eye causing the bothersome interference when viewing sustained viewing tasks such as watching television. The patch may then be removed when not in use.

References

1. Legge G, Parish DH, Luebker A, Wurm LEEH. Psychophysics of reading-XI Comparing color contrast. J Opt Soc Am. 1990;7(10):2002–10.
2. Wurm LH, Legge GE, Isenberg LM, Luebker A. Color improves object recognition in normal and low vision. J Exp Psychol Hum Percept Perform. 1993;19(4):899–911.
3. Brown B. Reading performance in low vision patients: relation to contrast and contrast sensitivity. Optom Vis Sci. 1981;
4. Legge GE, Rubin GS, Schleske MM. Contrast polarity effects in low vision reading. In: Low Vision. New York, NY: Springer New York; 1987. p. 288–307.
5. Rubin G, Legge G. Psychophysics of reading-VI The role of contrast in low vision. Vision Res. 1989;29(1):79–91.
6. RNIB. Accessibility of top 1,000 titles. www.rnib.org.uk (accessed 20.02.18)
7. Digre KB, Brennan K. Shedding light on photophobia. J Neuroophthalmol. 2012;32(1):68–81.
8. Eperjesi F, Fowler CW, Evans BJW. Do tinted lenses or filters improve visual performance in low vision? A review of the literature. Ophthalmic Physiol Opt. 2002;22(1):68–77.
9. Weale R. Retinal illumination and age. Light Res Technol. 1961;26(2):95–100.
10. Sörensen S, Brunnström G. Quality of light and quality of life: An intervention study among older people. Light Res Technol. 1995;27(2):113–8.
11. Cullinan T, Gould E, Silver J, Irvine D. Visual disability and home lighting. Lancet. 1979;313(8117):642–4.
12. Chartered Institution of Building Services Engineers (CIBSE). Lighting for people who are visually impaired. Soc Light Light. 2012;8(July):8–9.
13. Thomas Pocklington Trust. Lighting Solutions Guide. R Natl Inst Blind People. 2013;Edition 3.
14. Brunnström G, Sörensen S, Alsterstad K, Sjöstrand J. Quality of light and quality of life--the effect of lighting adaptation among people with low vision. Ophthalmic Physiol Opt. 2004;24:274–80.
15. Chartered Institution of Building Services Engineers (CIBSE). Light and lighting - Lighting of workplaces - Part 1: Indoor workplaces. BS EN 12464-1:2002 L. 2002.
16. Smith N, Carson G, Mallen EA. Lighting of Optometric Practices. Guidance Notes, The College of Optometrists. London; 2007. p. 1–11.
17. Carson GH. Eye Essentials: Environmental & Occupational Optometry. Doshi S, Harvey W, editors. Butterworth Heinemann, Elsevier; 2008. 67-76 p.

18. Haymes SA, Lee J. Effects of task lighting on visual function in age-related macular degeneration. Ophthalmic Physiol Opt. 2006;26(2):169–79.
19. Sheedy JE, Bailey I, Raasch T. Visual acuity and chart luminance. Am J Optom Physiol Opt. 1984;61(9):595–600.
20. Sloan LL. The photopic acuity-luminance function with special reference to parafoveal vision. Vision Res. 1968;8(7):901–11.
21. Sloan LL. Variation of acuity with luminance in ocular diseases and anomalies. Doc Ophthalmol. 1969;26(1):384–93.
22. Fosse P, Valberg A, Arnljot H. Retinal illuminance and the dissociation of letter and grating acuity in age-related macular degeneration. Vol. 78, Optometry and Vision Science. 2001. p. 162–8.
23. Adler G, Rottunda S. Older adults' perspectives on driving cessation. J Aging Stud. 2006;20(3):227–35.
24. Cummings RW, Whittaker SG, Watson GR, Budd JM. Scanning characters and reading with a central scotoma. Vol. 62, American Journal of Optometry and Physiological Optics. 1985. p. 833–43.
25. Crossland MD, Engel SA, Legge G. The preferred retinal locus in macula disease toward a consensus definition. 2011; Retina, Th:1–6.
26. Crossland MD, Culham LE, Kabanarou SA, Rubin GS. Preferred retinal locus development in patients with macular disease. Ophthalmology. 2005;112(9):1579–85.
27. Crossland MD, Culham LE, Rubin GS. Fixation stability and reading speed in patients with newly developed macular disease. Ophthalmic Physiol Opt. 2004;24(4):327–33.
28. Petre KL, Hazel C, Fine EM, Rubin GS. Reading with eccentric fixation is faster in inferior visual field than in left visual field. Optom Vis Sci. 2000;77(1):34–9.
29. Gaffney AJ, Margrain TH, Bunce C V., Binns AM. How effective is eccentric viewing training? A systematic literature review. Vol. 34, Ophthalmic and Physiological Optics. 2014. p. 427–37.
30. Whittaker SG, Budd J, Cummings RW. Eccentric fixation with macular scotoma. Investig Ophthalmol Vis Sci. 1988;29(2):268–78.
31. Gustafsson J, Inde K. The MoviText method : Efficient pre-optical reading training in persons with central visual field loss. Technol Disabil. 2004;6:211–21.
32. Stelmack J, Massof R, Stelmack T. Is there a standard of care for eccentric viewing training? J Rehabil Res Dev. 2004;41(5):729–38.
33. Smith HJH, Dickinson CCM, Cacho I, Reeves BC, Harper RA. A randomised controlled trial to determine the effectiveness of prism spectacles for patients with age-related macular degeneration. Arch of Opthal 2005; 123(8):1042–50.

34. Markowitz SN, Reyes S V., Sheng L. The use of prisms for vision rehabilitation after macular function loss: An evidence-based review. Acta Ophthalmol. 2013;91(3):207–11.
35. Beirne R, Meehan N. Does the E-Scoop lens improve visual performance in age-related macular degeneration? In: Optometry Tomorrow 2016 College of Optometrists[Conference contribution]. 2016.
36. Drasdo N, Murray IJ. A pilot study on the use of visual field expanders. Br J Physiol Opt. 1978;32:22–9.
37. Drasdo N. Visual field expanders. Am J Optom Physiol Opt. 1976;
38. Lowe J, Drasdo N. Patient's responses to retinitis pigmentosa. Optom Vis Sci. 1992;69(3):182–5.
39. Herse P. Retinitis pigmentosa: visual function and multidisciplinary management. Clin Exp Optom. 2005;88(5):335–50.
40. Cohen JM. An overview of enhancement techniques for peripheral field loss. J Am Optom Assoc. 1993;64(1):60–70.
41. Geruschat DR, Turano KA. Connecting research on retinitis pigmentosa to the practice of orientation and mobility. J Vis Impair Blind. 2002;96(2):69–85.
42. Nelles G, Esser J, Eckstein A, Tiede A, Gerhard H, Diener HC. Compensatory visual field training for patients with hemianopia after stroke. Neurosci Lett. 2001;306(3):189–92.
43. Peli E. Field expansion for homonymous hemianopia by optically induced peripheral exotropia. Optom Vis Sci. 2000;77(9):453–64.
44. Giorgi RG, Woods RL, Goldstein RB, Peli E, Bond T, Easton RD. Extended wearing trial of peripheral prism device for homonymous hemianopia (abstract). Investig Ophthalmol Vis Sci. 2004;45(5):1399.
45. Giorgi RG, Woods RL, Peli E. Clinical and laboratory evaluation of peripheral prism glasses for hemianopia. Optom Vis Sci. 2009;86(5):492–502.
46. Mort DJ, Malhotra P, Mannan SK, Rorden C, Pambakian A, Kennard C, et al. The anatomy of visual neglect. Brain. 2003;126(9):1986–97.

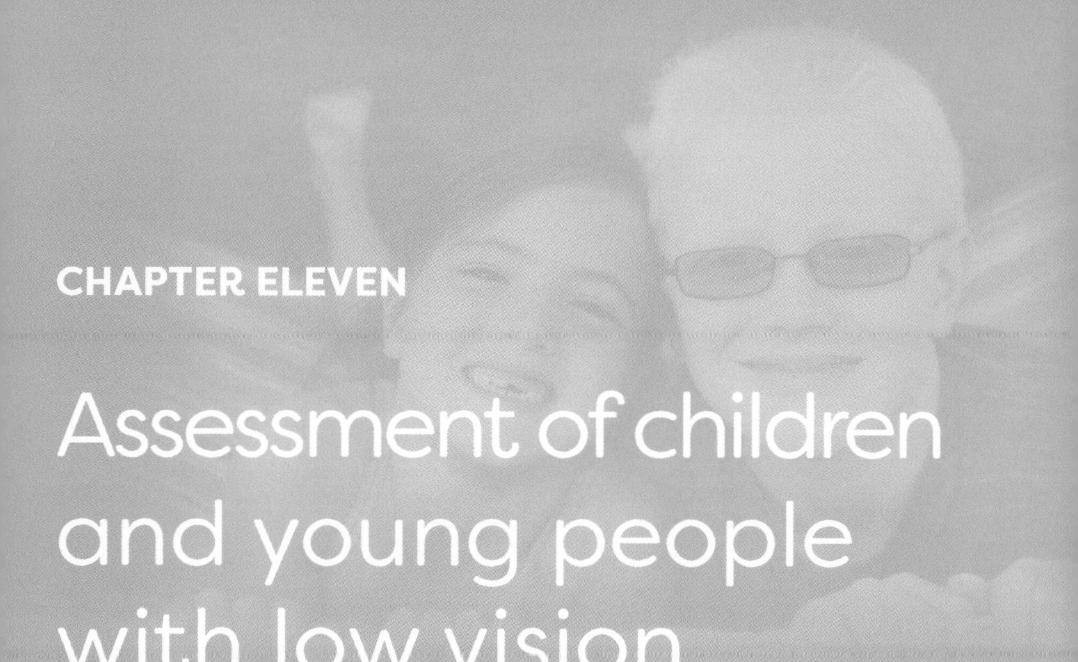

CHAPTER ELEVEN

Assessment of children and young people with low vision

Rasmeet K. Chadha MSc BSc Hons MCOptom
Oxford Eye Hospital, Oxford, UK.

> “The importance to us as a family to have full professional support in place before Lewis started his new school meant that the transition was less stressful for all of us as a family. He’s making great progress now.”
>
> **Adedayo, father of Lewis, aged 11**

Introduction

Paediatric low vision assessment and management can be thought of as a sub speciality within the field of low vision practice. This group of patients and their families require a multidisciplinary approach with the child at the centre of all decision making. The aim in the provision of paediatric low vision services is to ensure that the child is given every opportunity to achieve their maximum potential irrespective of their visual impairment.

For epidemiology of visual impairment see Chapter 1. In England and Wales the leading causes of childhood visual impairment in 2014-2015, were hereditary retinal dystrophies, disorders of the visual cortex and brain and nystagmus and other irregular eye movements.[1] There is now evidence that in lower income settings the traditional causes of visual impairment in children, infective and nutritional corneal opacities and congenital anomalies, are shifting to resemble the patterns seen in higher income settings.[2]

This chapter will cover the role of the multidisciplinary team in providing low vision provision. It will also cover, in detail, the low vision aid assessment.

The assessment of our younger patients encompasses a wide range of age groups. Where there is reference to **children** within this chapter the assumption will be made that **all age groups** are being discussed unless otherwise stated.

Similarly, where there is a reference to **parents** this also includes those who have guardianship or who may be the child or young person's representative.

The role of the multidisciplinary team

Ophthalmologist

The ophthalmologist is responsible for the initial diagnosis and for prescribing and undertaking any medical and surgical management. Referral to other medical professionals for joint working to confirm the diagnosis may be required such as to geneticists or paediatricians. Ensuring all available medical information is understood by the family and then shared with the multidisciplinary team will enable optimum rehabilitation for the child and their family.

Low vision practitioner

A number of suitably qualified individuals can perform this role individually or collectively. The list of individuals includes, but is not limited to, optometrists, dispensing opticians and orthoptists. They may be assisted by individuals who have had training in the provision of low vision therapy. The low vision assessment is a key part of paediatric low vision services provision and is covered in detail later in the chapter.

Education provision

There are a number of professionals who have a role in the education provision of a child with visual impairment. These individuals and their titles vary from country to country but can include the class teacher, a qualified teacher of children and young people with vision impairment, QTVI (an individual with a specialist qualification in supporting children with visual impairment), and teachers with additional qualifications in supporting children with special educational needs and disabilities. The roles of these individuals has become increasingly important as certainly in the developed world more children with visual impairment are now educated in mainstream schools.[3,4]

Rehabilitation services

There are many individuals who can provide this service either individually or collectively. These include, but are not limited to rehabilitation officers, orientation and mobility instructors, occupational therapists, or low vision practitioners with an additional qualification in rehabilitation. They may provide a range of services including teaching independent living skills, teaching communication skills and providing mobility training including long cane training.

Emotional support services

Visual impairment in childhood has lifelong implications for both the child and their family. Indeed, it affects the child's development, education, and the care given by families and professionals. It also shapes the adult the child will become, affecting employment and social prospects.[5] It is important to understand the lifetime of disability these children may endure and the impact that their visual impairment may have on family, friends and relationships. The effect of their disability may vary depending on the age they are or the environment they find themselves in and so the ongoing provision of low vision services and emotional support and social inclusion throughout childhood is essential. Emotional support in its broadest sense can be provided by any of the individuals described above or specialist counselling services may available through the general medical practitioner, or through charitable support services. Charitable support service may also provide local support groups for children and their families to meet one another.

Other professional groups

For a child with complex needs any of the above professionals may need to work closely with other professionals involved in supporting the child such as social workers, physiotherapists, speech and language therapists and health and educational professionals for the deaf.

The low vision assessment

The main focus of the assessment is naturally the child. However, parents, teachers, and other workers involved in supporting the child can be invited to attend or provide preliminary background information on the child to help ensure a more integrated approach. A pre-assessment questionnaire can be sent out to the parents ahead of the assessment to enable them to collect the views and thoughts of those individuals working and supporting the child.

History

Questions asked may include:

- Who is known to be currently supporting the child?
- What difficulties these individuals perceive the child to have in day to day activities?

- Have the parents been given sufficient information to understand their child's diagnosis?
- If appropriate is the child on a register of visual impairment or has this been offered to the family?

It is important that the low vision practitioner has a clear understanding of how much the parent and child understand the diagnosis to ensure that any information and advice that is given to them during or after the assessment continues on from their current level of understanding.

As when undertaking an eye examination, an accurate history and symptoms is a key part of the assessment. The practitioner must question proactively and involve the child and their parents in the history taking. The low vision assessment is often the start of an ongoing relationship with the practitioner, which can last for years. Continuity is really important and so wherever possible ensuring that the same practitioner sees the child for follow up appointments can help ensure the best ongoing integrated care.

History taking is an art and so it is important the child and parent feels comfortable with the process so that they can be open with any concerns or questions that they may have. Vision impairment in general affects four main functional areas:

- Orientation and mobility
- Communication
- Activities of daily living
- Sustained near vision tasks[6]

These areas should be covered in the history taking part of an assessment. However, as when conducting an eye examination it is important to question about general health and medications. Understanding the child's needs from a holistic perspective is important. An example of a structure that could be followed is given below:

Symptoms

It is unlikely that children and their parents will be able to answer direct questions such as what are the child's symptoms? Instead the practitioner may need to ask more specific and closed questions such as:

- Are there any problems with distance vision, near vision, glare, night vision or colour vision?
- How does lighting and glare affect the child's function?
- Does the child report headaches or asthenopia?

Be aware that a positive response to headaches or asthenopia (even in the absence of any reported visual difficulties) may suggest that the child is struggling with the visual demands placed upon them and may be the practitioner's only clue to the difficulties they experience. This may be because the child (particularly if a teenager) is reluctant to discuss their difficulties for fear of being given spectacles or optical aids that will make them look different or simply because the child, not knowing any different, has not appreciated the difficulties that their visual impairment has placed upon their visual system.

Use of spectacles, optical and electronic low vision aids

It is important to establish at the outset whether the child has been prescribed spectacles, whether they wear any prescribed spectacles and whether they use any low vision aids or glare protection aids. In the process of making a diagnosis, ensuring that the child is wearing the most appropriate refractive correction can be overlooked.

Teenagers may choose not to wear any prescribed spectacles or use any prescribed optical low vision aids as they are keen to ensure that they behave in the same way as their peers.

Younger children with nystagmus may not realise that they look over or under their spectacles when adopting an abnormal head posture to maximise vision by using their null position. Taking note of the way the spectacles fit, and when the patient or their parent reports that the spectacles are worn, is important.

Mainstream electronic technology has developed significantly in the last few years such that it can be used to enhance visual performance for children with visual impairment. For example, cameras on tablets and smartphones can be used to zoom in on the whiteboard in school or can be used to capture a scene, or document and then enlarge so that the patient can then access it more comfortably. Specialist electronic aids are still available and the child may already have access to such an aid at school.

School

Children spend a large proportion of their time in educational settings. It is important to spend time understanding the current school situation and the support that the child currently receives. Questions around ease of access to the whiteboard and to books/ worksheets are important.

- What sort of school does the child attend?
- Does the child receive any additional support from a qualified teacher for the visually impaired or related individual?
- Is the child forming the relationships/ friendships that would be expected for their age? It is known that vision can limit social interaction[6] and so care must be taken to establish if there are any perceived difficulties in this area.

Home

In conditions known to have a genetic predisposition the practitioner can establish whether other family members have a similar visual impairment. Having other family members with the same condition can mean that the family has a better understanding of the implications of the diagnosis but it can also mean that the child has heightened concerns about their diagnosis if they have seen the impact of the visual impairment on that individual.

- How has the diagnosis affected family and friend relationships and the emotional wellbeing of the child or young person and their parents?
- Have any modifications to the home environment been made already?

Mobility

- Can the child orientate and navigate well?
- Does the child have the level of independence that would be expected for their age?

Some children with visual impairment may be trained in the use of a long cane and may use this to improve their orientation and mobility particularly in unfamiliar environments. Some families may be interested in the option of a guide dog for when their child is older. It is worth taking time to explore issues surrounding mobility as well as any apprehensions that parents may have about their child developing the independence that would be expected of them at a given age so that appropriate solutions can be discussed.

Assessment of visual function

Visual acuity

It is important to realise that visual function does not necessarily correlate with visual acuity.[4] Accurate assessment of visual acuity is essential but equally an understanding of how this visual acuity and other clinical measures of vision translate into visual functioning is important to be able to understand how the child manages in their environment. For example, if a child is recorded as having distance visual acuity of 6/12 (logMAR 0.3), the parents and teachers will be interested in knowing what this means from a day to day point of view. Other professionals involved in supporting the child (such as qualified teachers for the visually impaired QTVI) can help the low vision practitioner translate clinical measures into a functional understanding.

The test chosen must be appropriate for the child's age and level of understanding. When measuring distance vision, for school age children, the use of logMAR charts as described in Chapter 3 may be appropriate. There are specific logMAR charts for children available, such as Kay pictures, Keeler logMAR crowded test or Lea symbols (Figure 11.1).

Near vision assessment is probably one of the most important parts of the low vision assessment. This is because vision 'up close' is where most of the child's day to day activities are focused (reading, writing, computer, eating, seeing

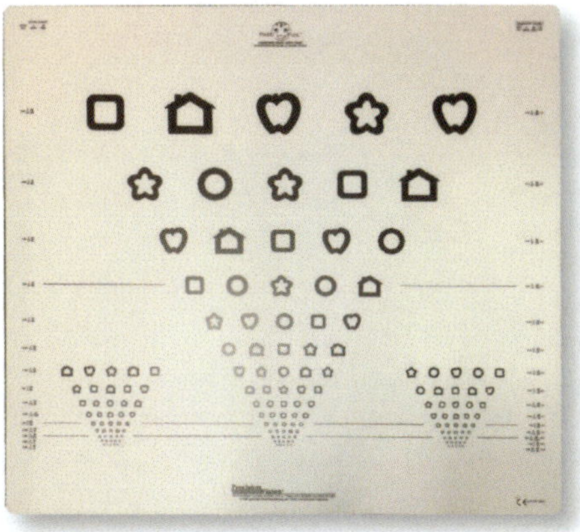

Figure 11.1 A logMAR insert for the ETDRS chart consisting of Lea Symbols.

faces of family and friends). Children with visual impairment often hold reading material very close to benefit from relative distance magnification (objects appear twice as big if held twice as close, Chapter 5). Therefore it is important to measure the child's near vision at their preferred reading distance and record this clearly in the notes.

It is also important to establish if any difficulty reading is due to visual impairment or the child's ability to read. The Maclure reading test type for children (Figure 11.2) is very useful from this point of view. It has a series of pages that provide text of varying sizes that are specific to a given age. Hence it can assist the practitioner in establishing whether poor reading ability is because of the visual impairment or the child's reading ability. Care must be taken to ensure the concept of acuity reserve is taken into account. Refer to Chapter 5 when translating clinical measures of near vision into expected functional outcomes.

Contrast sensitivity

An appreciation of contrast sensitivity can help the low vision practitioner appreciate the functional vision of the child. In a normally functioning visual system there is a predictable relationship between visual acuity and contrast sensitivity.[7] This relationship breaks down for those with visual impairment. For example, two children, both with VA of 6/12 (logMAR 0.3) may have very different contrast sensitivity functions and so may orientate very differently from one another in the real world.

The test charts described in Chapter 3 may be appropriate to test older children but for younger children there are specific charts such as the Hiding Heidi low contrast test.

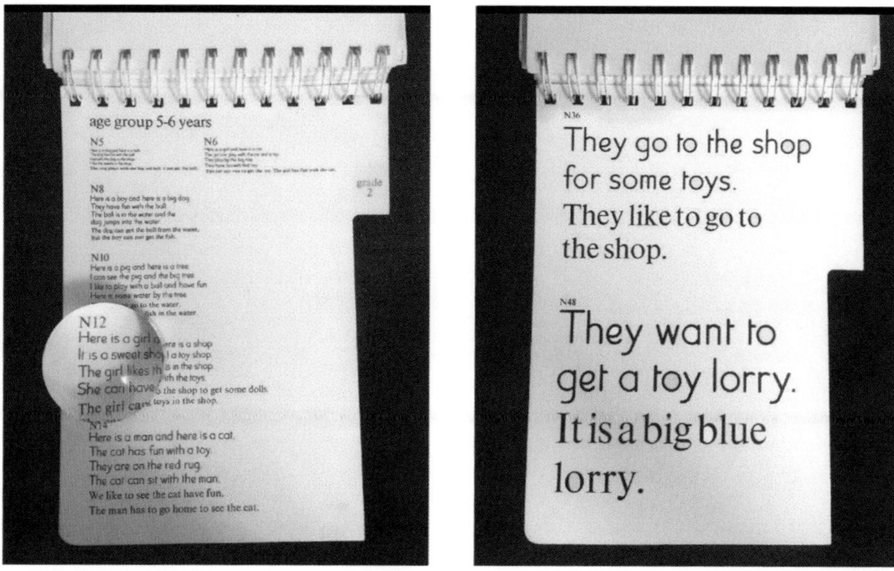

Figure 11.2 The Maclure reading test type for children is designed to differentiate between children's ability to see and their ability to read. Each age has been giving a grade (1-7) so that even if a child's reading ability is not equal to the average age, it can still be recorded by the grade number. The test is based upon the Ladybird Keywords reading scheme (www.penguin.co.uk/ladybird) using school script, which is a simplified type written without serifs. Within each grade, print size ranges from N5 to N48.

Visual Fields

Measurement of visual fields can be challenging in younger children but an understanding of the visual fields can be really valuable as visual field loss can affect orientation and mobility. It can also influence advice given for day to day activities such as placement in the classroom. For example, a child with a right homonymous hemianopia could be advised to sit on the right hand side in the classroom so that most of the classroom activities occur in their seeing field.

In younger children, confrontation fields may be the most useful way to assess gross peripheral fields. Older children, age 6 and over, may manage Goldmann perimetry which can be an invaluable way to assess peripheral visual fields, however, the perimeter is not readily available. There are now computerised versions of the Goldmann perimeter available such as the Octopus perimeter. Standard static perimetry can be used to assess visual fields in older children and can be especially useful when central field loss is suspected, for example, in macular pathology.

Colour Vision

Assessment of colour vision is important to interpret anticipated difficulties at home and at school. For example, children with colour vision loss may have difficulty reading maps in geography lessons or interpreting science experiment results.

It is important to consider not only congenital colour vision defects but also acquired loss as a result of the pathology that results in the visual impairment. For acquired loss it may be useful to re-test colour vision over time to provide up to date information on colour vision and its likely impact in day-to-day activities.

Testing of colour vision in patients with visual impairment can be challenging as the limitation(s) of visual acuity and contrast sensitivity can make undertaking the test difficult or at times impossible.

Testing using for example Ishihara's test for colour deficiency, tests for red/green colour vision deficiency or a similar test can be an acceptable choice of screening test. Other tests of value in the paediatric population are the Farnsworth D-15 and HRR (Hardy, Rand and Rittler) Pseudoisochromatic Plates.

Refraction and accommodation

Accurate refraction and appropriate prescribing are essential in the context of paediatric low vision work to ensure that the child is given the best possible opportunity to maximise their visual functioning. Sadly, uncorrected refractive error remains a common cause of visual impairment in the developed world.[8]

Retinoscopy (and arguably cycloplegic retinoscopy) should form the first part of the refraction routine as it can provide information that may be missed if just a subjective refraction is performed, e.g. latent hyperopia or the presence of visually significant lens opacities. Refraction can be difficult in children with vision impairment but similar strategies used when refracting adults with vision impairment can be employed. For example, binocular refraction can be undertaken for those with nystagmus which increases in amplitude on monocular occlusion.

Children with visual impairment often use relative distance magnification to attain better near vision than would be expected from the measurement of their distance vision by exerting high levels of accommodation. It is therefore, important, to accurately assess the accommodative function of the child with visual impairment. Accommodation can be measured subjectively using for example, the RAF-rule or can be measured objectively using dynamic retinoscopy.

Accommodative weakness is known to occur in children with certain conditions, such as those with Down's syndrome or cerebral palsy.[7] Therefore, these groups of children may require positive near additions or bifocals to maximise their near vision and/or may require near optical aids earlier than their peers with normal accommodative function.

Prescribing

Optical aids

The prescribing of optical aids requires an understanding of not only the visual capabilities and task requirements of the child but also the child's additional needs and social situation. For example, a child with cerebral palsy may have problems with manual dexterity making handling of a hand magnifier more difficult.

Prescribing spectacles in the context of amblyopia or refractive management is the same as for any other child. However, there are some additional considerations when prescribing spectacles for children with visual impairment. For example, the correction of lower refractive errors than would have been considered in children with normal vision may result in improved near vision due to enhancement of accommodation. Children who are myopic may actually sustain better near vision if allowed to read unaided due to the reduced accommodative demand in this situation. Children with visual impairment can have high refractive errors and so care must be taken when choosing a spectacle frame to ensure it is fit for purpose.

Contact lenses can be a safe, practical and appropriate solution for some children with visual impairment. For example, children with high myopia may see better in contact lenses than in spectacles. Children who are tactile defensive (have heightened sensitivity to touch or tactile input) may have difficulty adapting to spectacle wear and may initially prefer to wear contact lenses, providing their parent is proficient in the insertion and removal of contact lenses.

Before prescribing optical low vision aids it is important to establish the goals and to ensure that these are realistic. The goals can be set following the discussion during history and symptoms as well as information which may be gathered in the pre-assessment questionnaire. It is important to be realistic at this stage, for example, a child who can only read N48 size font will be unlikely to be able to fluently read N5 size font with a conventional optical aid. This child may rely on text enlargement, electronic aid provision and / or Braille. Optical aids can be prescribed for distance vision and for near vision. Optical aids for near vision are only usually needed when accommodative reserve does not match the task requirements. Distance aids can be prescribed as soon as a need is established for them but in reality children younger than age 6-7 may find the focussing of monoculars or binoculars difficult.

There are a number of near optical aids available and generally these fall into the same groups as for when prescribing for adults. This list includes: high reading additions, hand or pocket magnifiers, stand magnifiers and bar or brightfield magnifiers. The superior light gathering properties and ease of use of the brightfield magnifier makes it a popular choice in the paediatric group (Figure 11.3).

Distance aids include monoculars and binoculars. The choice as to whether a monocular or binocular is prescribed can be in part down to patient preference but the practitioner should take into consideration the cause of the vision impairment when helping the patient to make a decision. For example, patients with nystagmus may prefer a binocular as using a monocular may exacerbate the nystagmus and therefore result in reduced visual function.

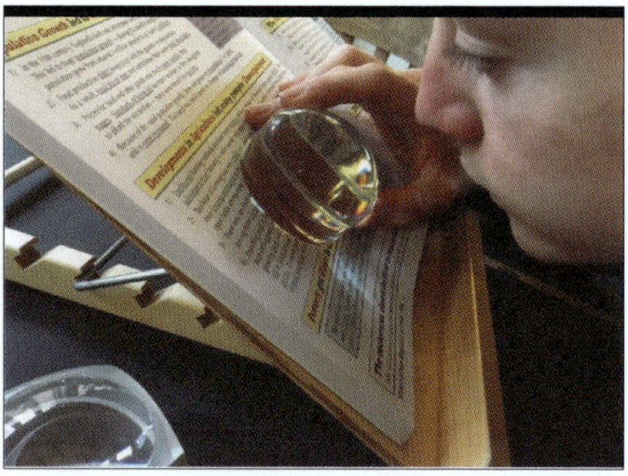

Figure 11.3 The patient is using a dome magnifier to assist with a school book. Children tend to work close to the page and many benefit from using a reading slope within the school setting to assist with posture.

Non-optical aids

Non-optical aids can be used in isolation or in conjunction with optical aids. There are a wide variety of non-optical aids available to help with all aspects of activities of daily living and many of these are similar to those used by adult patients with visual impairment. Examples of non-optical aids that are particularly useful in the paediatric group include text enlargement at school, the use of black fibre tip pens when writing, sloping desks at school to ensure posture is not compromised by a close working distance and enhanced local lighting.

Children in the early years of school, with mild/moderate visual impairment, may not require regular text enlargement as print size is naturally large and when combined with relative distance magnification they can manage well. However, as they progress through the school years and as print size reduces and as their accommodative reserve reduces they may need regular text enlargement and may need to use optical near aids.

Electronic aids

The area of electronic aid provision has developed exponentially in recent years as described above. Electronic aids have their place alongside optical and non-optical aids and often the well-adjusted child with visual impairment will use a combination of optical, non-optical and electronic aids at home and at school to maximise their visual potential.

Tints and glare management

Children with visual impairment can suffer with photophobia in the same way as adults with visual impairment. Consideration as to the most appropriate way to manage this must be given and different solutions may be needed for home than for school. For example, the windows in the classroom may prove to be a glare source for the child with visual impairment and it may be appropriate to consider the child's position in the classroom to minimise the effect of this glare. Photochromic lenses can be a good solution for the older child but those with severe photophobia (e.g. achromatopsia) may find that that even in the darkened state that photochromic lenses do not provide enough protection from the glare source. In cases of severe photophobia it may be appropriate to consider a 5% tint along with side shields on the spectacles (Figure 11.4) and a brimmed hat for when outdoors.

Communication

Rahi et al reported parents valued most the information that they received from their child's ophthalmologist and also from clinical staff in the ophthalmology department.[9] Clear communication at the point of diagnosis and thereafter is essential.

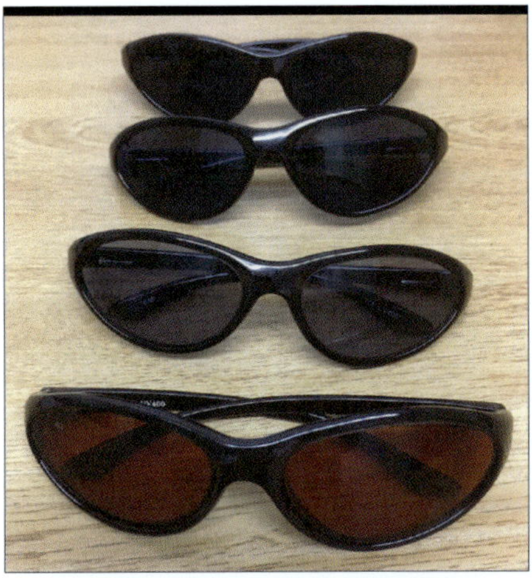

Figure 11.4 A selection of paediatric wrap-around plano sunglasses for children from the extensive *NoIR Low Vision Filter System*. 'Fitover' filter spectacles are also available for those children who require a spectacle prescription.

The diagnosis is usually given by an ophthalmologist but the low vision practitioner has a key role in ensuring that the parent and child (where appropriate) have a clear understanding of the diagnosis. Parents and older children may go through a bereavement process as described in Chapter 12. The low vision practitioner has a role in supporting the family through this process and signposting to emotional support/counselling services when appropriate.

Paediatric low vision provision requires a multidisciplinary approach. Communication between all professionals and also with parents and with the child (when they are old enough) is crucial in ensuring that the needs of the child are appropriately met. Solutions to concerns raised during history taking need to be clearly discussed during or at the end of the assessment with the child and parent. The solutions proposed by the practitioner have to be acceptable to the child and the parent for them to implement them outside of the testing room environment.

It is important to have the child and their parent on board when dispensing an optical low vision aid. The child and their parent need to be clear about the anticipated use of the aid. This two way dialogue can help ensure acceptance and use of the low vision aid.

It is important to regularly follow up children with visual impairment, especially at times of transition such as when changing school or when moving into further or higher education.

As the child moves through school the demands on their visual system change and so they may need a change to the advice given or the aids dispensed. Also, teenage children may begin to reject the optical low vision aids that they readily used when they were younger. The low vision practitioner needs to be receptive to this and have alterative low vision aids or advice on non-optical or electronic aids available for consideration.

Report writing

Lennon et al reported a high level of satisfaction amongst parents who received written reports following their child's low vision appointment.[10] The report can serve not only as an aide memoire to parents or guardians but can be used by the other professionals supporting the child to ensure that the recommendations made and advice given is still appropriate.

The report can include as much or as little information as the practitioner thinks is useful. It may include:

- A detailed explanation of diagnosis.
- An outline of visual function and an explanation of the likely functional impact of this visual function. For example " the recorded visual acuity of 6/12 means that objects need to be 3x as big or 3x as close to be seen as clearly as normally sighted peers."
- Information on the spectacles advised or glare protection discussed.
- Information on optical low vision aids dispensed and the anticipated use for these aids as well as any advice given on non-optical or electronic aids.
- Information on planned follow up and contact details for the practitioner.

Summary

Paediatric low vision provision is a multidisciplinary process. Long term follow up of patients is essential to ensure that the changing visual needs are addressed throughout their childhood and adolescent years. Care must be taken when prescribing spectacles and when dispensing optical low vision aids to ensure that they meet the requirements of the patient and help maximise visual potential. Good communication with the child and parent from the point of diagnosis is essential. Written reports following the low vision assessment can be an invaluable source of information for all involved in the care and support of the child.

References

1. Bunce C, Zekite A, Wormald R, Bowman R. Is there evidence that the yearly numbers of children newly certified with sight impairment in England and Wales has increased between 1999/2000 and 2014/2015? A cross-sectional study. BMJ Open. 2017;7(9).
2. Solebo AL, Teoh L, Rahi J. Epidemiology of blindness in children. Arch Dis Child. 2017;102(9):853–7.
3. Royal National Institute of Blind People (RNIB). Educational provision for blind and partially sighted children and young people in England. London. 2007;
4. Lawrence L, Wilson M. Paediatric Low Vision. In: Wilson M.,Trivedi R., Saunders R. (eds) Paediatric Ophthalmology. Springer, Berlin, Heidelberg. 2009.
5. Rahi JS, Cable N. Severe visual impairment and blindness in the UK. Lancet. 2003;362:1359–65.
6. World Health Organisation. Management of low vision in children. Report of a WHO consultation, Bangkok. WHO/PBL/9337. 1992;8–10.
7. Hyvarinen L, Jacob N. What and how does this child see?, Finland, Pub: VISTEST Ltd. 2011. Chp 4.
8. Nelson B, Olitsky S. Harley's Pediatric Ophthalmology, Philadelphia, Lippincott Williams and Wilkins Ed6. 2015.
9. Rahi JS, Manaras I, Barr K. Information sources and their use by parents of children with ophthalmic disorders. Investig Ophthalmol Vis Sci. 2003;44(6):2457–60.
10. Lennon J, Harper R, Lloyd C, Biswas S. Usefulness of post-assessment reports in a paediatric low vision clinic: A questionnaire survey of parents and education professionals. Ophthalmic Physiol Opt. 2008;28(3):247–52.

CHAPTER TWELVE

The Impact of Visual Impairment and Rehabilitation

Dr Keziah Latham BSc PhD FCOptom Prof Cert LV FHEA
Anglia Ruskin University, Cambridge, UK.

> “Rehabilitation is a journey beyond light and darkness. Professional intervention can enhance existing and teach new skills, increasing confidence and maximising independence.”
>
> **Rebecca Scott, Rehabilitation Service Coordinator, Vista, UK.**

The Impact of Visual Impairment and Rehabilitation

Impairment, activity limitation, participation restriction

Visual impairment is the result of a disease affecting the function of the eye, and the level of impairment can be assessed by measuring visual function, as outlined in previous chapters. Such impairment results in limitations in the activities (execution of a task or action by an individual) that a person with a visual impairment can undertake or complete, and potentially then also restrictions to that person's participation in society (involvement in a life situation). For example, someone with macular degeneration will have reduced visual acuity (impairment), which impacts on their ability to read (activity limitation). This may affect their ability to gain or remain in employment or to continue valued hobbies (participation restriction). The World Health Organisation[1] has outlined nine domains that cover the areas in which activities and participation can be considered in its International Classification of Functioning, Disability and Health (ICF) (Table 12.1). It is also useful to consider a tenth domain of emotional health.[2]

To reduce or prevent activity limitations and participation restrictions that result from visual impairment may require changes to 'personal factors' (how the person views their situation, or aids that a person might use on an individual basis), or to 'environmental factors' (the physical, social, and attitudinal environment in which people live and conduct their lives).

The term 'disability' is now used as an umbrella term that covers impairments, activity limitations and participation restrictions. The idea of this terminology is to get away from categorising people as 'healthy' or 'disabled', but to acknowledge that everyone can have decrements in health that cause them some form of disability.[1] The term 'handicap' is no longer used.

Quality of life

There are several terms that will be come across when considering the overall impact of vision loss on the quality of a person's life.[3,4] Quality of life (QoL), is defined as 'an evaluation of all aspects of our lives, including, for example,

Table 12.1 Domains of the WHO ICF[1].

Domain	Examples
Learning and applying knowledge	Reading and writing
General tasks and demands	Routine tasks such as dealing with personal administration
Communication	Including use of telephones and computers
Mobility	Including walking, and use of transport
Self-care	Such as personal hygiene, eating and drinking
Domestic life	Including household chores and shopping
Interpersonal interactions and relationships	With different groups of people from strangers to family members
Major life areas	Including work and education
Community, social and civic life	Such as hobbies, sports and social events

where we live, how we live, and how we play. It encompasses such life factors as family circumstances, finances, housing and job satisfaction'.[3] A related concept is health-related quality of life (HR-QoL), defined as: 'Personal health status. HR-QoL usually refers to aspects of our lives that are dominated or significantly influenced by our mental or physical well-being'.[3] A further relevant concept is vision-related quality of life (VR-QoL), where assessment of functional vision (as opposed to visual function) is considered.[5] To try and capture such perceived difficulties with quality of life domains, patient reported outcomes measures (PROMs) in the form of questionnaires are often used. There are a large number of questionnaires available including many designed to address specific ophthalmic concerns.[6] Commonly used examples include the National Eye Institute Visual Function Questionnaire (NEI-VFQ),[7] The Impact of Vision Impairment instrument (IVI),[8] and the Low Vision Quality of Life questionnaire (LVQOL).[9]

Assessment of rehabilitation needs

The aim of rehabilitation is to reduce the activity limitations and participation restrictions that result from visual impairment by addressing either personal or environmental factors. Given that visual loss can have such a profound effect on people, the rehabilitation services that people need can be wide ranging and cover all the different domains of the WHO ICF. The low vision practitioner has an important role in recognising patients' needs for different areas of rehabilitation and in signposting on to services that go beyond the practitioner's own remit. Patients themselves often do not know what sort of help they could benefit from, or what services are available.

Areas that patients may need help with are covered by the terms 'activities of daily living' (ADLs) and 'instrumental activities of daily living' (IADLs). ADLs refer to basic necessary routine activities such as eating, bathing and dressing, whereas IADLs cover activities that are not fundamental but allow independent living, such as doing housework, shopping, or preparing meals. Determining all of a patient's rehabilitation needs due to vision loss can be complex and time consuming. Practitioners will use case history to explore with a patient the main difficulties they have resulting from their vision impairment that need addressing through rehabilitation. Questionnaires have also been designed that can be used to systematically determine rehabilitation needs. These include the Veterans Affairs Low-Vision Visual Functioning Questionnaire (LV VFQ-48),[10] Activity Inventory,[11] and Participation and Activity Inventory (PAI).[12] Such questionnaires ask about the difficulty perceived by the person in undertaking various specific visually related tasks, nested under broader areas of need such as 'reading' or 'mobility'. Although they may be time consuming to administer, they have the potential to identify more of a patient's rehabilitation needs than a case history approach.[13]

Rehabilitation services are provided in many different settings by a range of service providers and professionals, with personnel from health care, social care, and the voluntary sector likely to be involved. Many services will accept self-referrals, so that referral can be achieved by the practitioner giving contact details of an organisation to their patient. Some services may require more formal referral through health or social care systems, or be triggered by visual impairment registration.

In the following sections, key areas of impact of visual impairment in terms of psychological wellbeing and orientation and mobility are discussed, going beyond those needs already considered with regard to optical aids. Many other areas of rehabilitation will also be relevant to patients (for example, finance and benefits, employment, travel, and sport), but appropriate information on these more specific areas will be location dependent and so is not considered in detail here .

Psychological impact of visual impairment

Acquired visual loss can be considered a form of bereavement, and someone who loses their vision must mourn its loss in order to be able to move on in their life with a new status as a person with a visual impairment. For someone with chronic and changing visual loss, this may be an ongoing process as vision deteriorates. Kübler-Ross[14] presented a theoretical model of grieving, consisting of a number of potential stages. These stages can be helpful to consider in terms of how they may influence a practitioner's communication with people with a visual impairment.

Shock

When someone is diagnosed with irreversible or untreatable sight loss, a common response is that of shock. A patient who is in shock will be unlikely to be able to take in much further information about their condition or its prognosis. Practitioners who are involved in providing diagnoses would be advised to provide crucial information in a form that the patient can take away with them for later reference (remembering that if information is given in printed form to use a print size that can be seen), and / or for the patient to be able to access information again at a future date once the diagnosis has had a chance to sink in. For practitioners working with patients at a point after diagnosis, it is always well worth checking what a patient's understanding of their diagnosis is: although they may have been given excellent information at the time, little of it may have been retained, making a follow up conversation very valuable.

Denial

Patients may go through a stage of denial regarding the severity of their visual loss or its irreversibility. The practitioner may come across this in patients who attend multiple practitioners in the hope of receiving a different diagnosis, or who are convinced that 'they just need stronger glasses'. It is important to be realistic with such patients and not to give them false hope of a miraculous improvement in their vision.

Equally, it will be difficult for patients who are not able to acknowledge their visual loss to seek out or to attend low vision rehabilitation services. Practitioners can still make patients aware of services that are available for future reference, even if they are not in a position to access those services at that point.

Anger / grief

Grief and anger can appear in a similar way. Patients need to grieve for their lost vision, and may dwell on what they cannot do now that they could before. Frustration with functional loss can lead to anger, which may be directed internally, with the patient perhaps blaming themselves for their loss of vision. Anger can also be directed externally, including at the practitioner for not being able to do more to resolve the problem.

Depression

Depression is extremely common in people with visual impairment, with studies suggesting that up to a half of patients with a visual impairment how significant symptoms of depression, but with many not receiving treatment for depression.[15] Depression may be driven in part by the patient's lack of ability to do desired tasks, so the eyecare practitioner's role in providing low vision aids to help with achieving such tasks can be valuable in improving mental health.

The eyecare practitioner can also assist by identifying patients for whom visual impairment is causing distress, and referring them on for treatment by an appropriate professional. It can be obvious from a patient's presentation or case history that they are struggling with the emotional consequences of vision loss, but practitioners can also ask two questions suggested for identification of depression in patients with chronic physical health problems, [16] which are:

- During the last month, have you often been bothered by feeling down, depressed or hopeless?
- During the last month, have you often been bothered by having little interest or pleasure in doing things?

If a patient answers 'yes' to either question, they should be referred to a professional competent to perform a mental health assessment, such as their general medical practitioner.

Other resources providing emotional support, rather than specific treatment for depression, may be available such as counselling through peer group support or self-management programmes,[17,18] befriending services, and informal support through social events of charitable organisations. These emotional support services can be invaluable even if a patient does not screen positively for depression, as 'having someone to talk to' is a key need for many people with vision loss.[19,20]

Remember also to consider those who attend appointments with a visually impaired person, it has been found that up to a third of caregivers also have significant levels of depressive symptoms.[21]

Acceptance

Someone who has 'accepted' their visual loss has come to terms with their new identity as a person with a visual impairment, and are much more likely to accept interventions such as low vision aids. They may also be less concerned about cosmetic aspects such as whether low vision aids make them look 'different' or draw attention to them. This does not mean that low vision aids or other services should not be offered to patients who are obviously at a different stage in coming to terms with their visual loss. It may be that patients at an earlier stage are not yet ready to accept assistance, but by making patients aware of what is available, they will be more aware of the options and the benefits of re-accessing services when they are ready.

Many factors have been suggested to affect how well and how quickly someone comes to terms with their visual loss. Factors that have generally been found to be associated with better adjustment to visual loss include acceptance of vision loss as being irreversible, the use of problem-solving approaches to coping with difficulties, a belief that the individual has control over their life (internal locus of control), and good social support.[22]

Impact of visual impairment on mobility

Orientation and mobility training

Orientation (working out where you are) and mobility (getting to where you want to be) can be very difficult for those with visual impairment, particularly if peripheral visual field is restricted, and can easily lead to loss of independence in travel.[23] Ocular conditions resulting in impaired peripheral field include those which result in general constriction of the field (e.g. retinitis pigmentosa, glaucoma), or those which result in hemianopic type field restriction (e.g. stroke).

Orientation and mobility training aims to give users more confident access to their environment. Training may include practicing specific routes, using public transport, and / or using mobility aids. Symbol canes, or short white folding canes, can be provided as an indicator of visual impairment (Figure 12.1). A white cane with red bands indicates that the user is also hearing impaired. Guide canes and long canes can be used to avoid obstacles and travel independently (Figure 12.2). Training in their use is required, and is often provided by a rehabilitation officer. Guide dogs can also aid in independent travel, and electronic devices and apps that use global positioning systems (GPS) and echolocation to aid in orientation and mobility are also becoming more widely available.

Falls

Visual impairment is an independent risk factor for falling, alongside many other issues including increasing age, taking multiple medications, mobility limitations, and home or environmental hazards.[24] It is important to reduce the risk of falls given their high personal and societal cost – not only is there a considerable health care cost, but also potential distress, loss of confidence, loss of independence and increased mortality.[25]

Reducing the risk of falls is a multifactorial process that needs to take the relevance of all risk factors into account. Interventions should include home hazard assessment, strength and balance training, medication review, and visual assessment.[25]

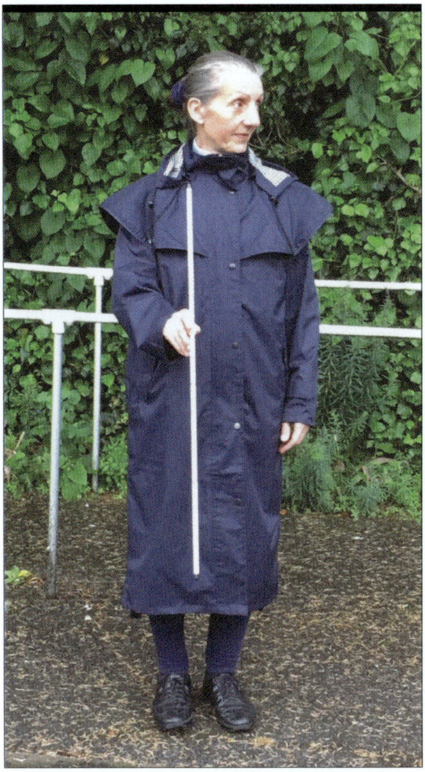

Figure 12.1 A symbol cane is used to indicate visual impairment.

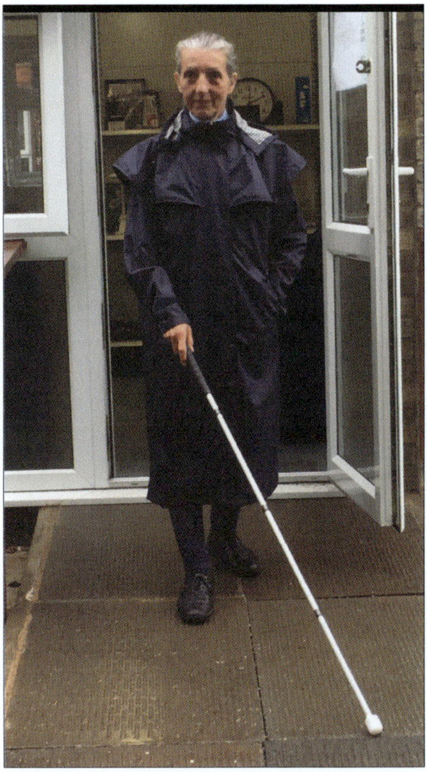

Figure 12.2 Using a long cane often requires several sessions of training from rehabilitation teams.

Minimising visual impairment through vision assessment and optimising refractive correction is important. However, care needs to be given to the form of spectacles dispensed. It is known that multifocal (bifocal or progressive addition lens) wearers are less stable and more likely to fall than single vision spectacle wearers.[26] It has therefore been suggested that patients at greater risk of falling, or who have previously fallen, should be recommended single vision spectacles, at least when out and about outside the home.[26] It is advised not to move patients at risk of falls from single vision to multifocal correction. Existing multifocal wearers may well be resistant to moving to single vision correction, with a loss of convenience in their spectacle correction. For these patients, minimising changes in lens design and giving advice on caution while adapting to refractive change would be appropriate.

Overview of rehabilitation services

There are many barriers to patients accessing rehabilitation services. Patients may not know what sort of help they could benefit from, or what services are available.[27,28] Even if a patient knows what type of service they would like to access, having visual impairment makes seeking out information about services a challenge, so eyecare practitioners are ideally placed to refer or signpost patients to relevant services. The most valuable management that a practitioner can make is often to signpost patients to services that go beyond their own remit.

The way that low vision services are organised vary dramatically according to location. Only general information can therefore be given here, and practitioners are advised to determine what services are available in their local area and how patients can be referred to them.

Many different professionals are involved in providing rehabilitation. Services may be provided by eyecare practitioners (e.g. optometrists, dispensing opticians, orthoptists), health care practitioners (e.g. doctors, nurses, counsellors), social care practitioners (e.g. rehabilitation officers, social workers) and professionals within the voluntary sector. These professionals may work in stand-alone services, or in multidisciplinary service provision.

Rehabilitation services have been shown to have generally beneficial effects on functional ability, such as the ability to read smaller print, but there is less evidence of impact on overall quality of life.[28,29] Although combining different elements of rehabilitation within a multidisciplinary service seems preferable,[30,31] there is to date a lack of good quality evidence on the effectiveness of services and the best ways to provide rehabilitative care .[28,29]

Summary

Visual impairment has a significant impact on a person's functional ability and emotional state. The rehabilitation needs of people with a visual impairment are therefore often wide ranging, covering services beyond the scope of the eyecare practitioner. However, the eyecare practitioner has an important role in identifying patients' potential needs, and signposting them to other services and service providers. Since service models and availability vary widely, it is important for practitioners to identify relevant services that are local to themselves and establish how patients can be referred to these services.

References

1. World Health Organization. The International Classification of Functioning, Disability and Health (ICF). Geneva. 2001;18:237.
2. Bruijning JE, Nispen R van, van Nispen R, Verstraten P, van Rens G. A Dutch ICF version of the Activity Inventory: results from focus groups with visually impaired persons and experts. Ophthalmic Epidemiol. 2010;17(6):366–77.
3. Patrick DL, Guyatt GH, Acquadro C. Cochrane handbook for systematic reviews of interventions version 5.1.0 [updated March 2011]. In: in Higgins, J P T & Green, S (eds) The Cochrane Collaboration. 2011. p. Chapter 17.
4. Taylor DJ, Hobby AE, Binns AM, Crabb DP. How does age-related macular degeneration affect real-world visual ability and quality of life? A systematic review. BMJ Open. 2016;6(12).
5. de Boer MR, Moll AC, de Vet HCW, Terwee CB, Völker-Dieben HJM, van Rens GHMB. Psychometric properties of vision-related quality of life questionnaires: a systematic review. Ophthalmic Physiol Opt. 2004;24(4):257–73.
6. Khadka J, McAlinden C, Pesudovs K. Quality assessment of ophthalmic questionnaires: review and recommendations. Optom Vis Sci. 2013;90(8):720–44.
7. Mangione CM, Lee PP, Pitts J, Gutierrez PR, Berry S, Hays RD. Psychometric properties of the National Eye Institute Visual Function Questionnaire (NEI-VFQ). Arch Ophthalmol. 1998 Nov 1;116(11):1496.

8. Weih LM, Hassell JB, Keeffe J. Assessment of the impact of vision impairment. Investig Ophthalmol Vis Sci. 2002;43(4):927–35.

9. Wolffsohn JS, Cochrane AL. Design of the low vision quality-of-life questionnaire (LVQOL) and measuring the outcome of low-vision rehabilitation. Am J Ophthalmol. 2000;130(6):793–802.

10. Stelmack JA, Tang XC, Reda DJ, Rinne S, Mancil RM, Massof RW. Outcomes of the Veterans Affairs Low Vision Intervention Trial (LOVIT). Arch Ophthalmol. 2008;126(5):608–17.

11. Massof RW, Ahmadian L, Grover LL, Deremeik JT, Goldstein JE, Rainey C, et al. The Activity Inventory: an adaptive visual function questionnaire. Optom Vis Sci. 2007;84(8):763–74.

12. van Leeuwen LM, Rainey L, Kef S, van Rens GHMB, van Nispen RMA. Investigating rehabilitation needs of visually impaired young adults according to the International Classification of Functioning, Disability and Health. Acta Ophthalmol. 2015;93(7):642–50.

13. Bruijning JE, van Nispen R, Knol D, van Rens G. Low vision rehabilitation plans comparing two intake methods. Optom Vis Sci. 2012;89(2):203–14.

14. Kübler-Ross E. On death and dying. New York: Macmillan Books. Touchstone Books, New York; 1969.

15. Nollett CL, Bray N, Bunce C V., Casten RJ, Edwards RT, Hegel MT, et al. High prevalence of Untreated depression in patients accessing low vision services. Ophthalmology. 2016;123(2):440–1.

16. National Institute for Health and Care Excellence (NICE). CG91 - Depression in adults with a chronic physical health problem: recognition and management. London; 2009.

17. Latham K. Evaluation of an emotional support service for the visually impaired. Optom Vis Sci. 2013;90(8):836–42.

18. Rees G, Xie J, Chiang PP, Larizza MF, Marella M, Hassell JB, et al. A randomised controlled trial of a self-management programme for low vision implemented in low vision rehabilitation services. Patient Educ Couns. 2015;98(2):174–81.

19. Pybis J, Thurston M, Dennison CM, Broom M, Miller A. The nature of emotional support and counselling provision for people with sight loss in the United Kingdom. Br J Vis Impair. 2016;34(2):169–78.

20. Royal National Institute of Blind People (RNIB). Sight loss : What we needed to know. U.K. Vision Strategy. London; 2016. p. 1–48.

21. Bambara JK, Owsley C, Wadley V, Martin R, Porter C, Dreer LE. Family caregiver social problem-solving abilities and adjustment to caring for a relative with vision loss. Investig Ophthalmol Vis Sci. 2009;50(4):1585–92.

22. Senra H, Barbosa F, Ferreira P, Vieira CR, Perrin PB, Rogers H, et al. Psychologic adjustment to irreversible vision voss in adults: A Systematic review. Ophthalmology. 2015;122(4):851–61.

23. Turano KA, Broman AT, Bandeen-Roche K, Munoz B, Rubin GS, West S. Association of visual field loss and mobility performance in older adults: Salisbury Eye Evaluation Study. Optom Vis Sci. 2004;81(5):298–307.

24. Thomas Pocklington Trust. Falls in older people with sight loss: a review of emerging research and key action points. Thomas Pocklington Trust. London; 2013.

25. National Institute for Health and Care Excellence (NICE). CG161 - Falls in older people : assessing risk and pre prevention. London; 2013.

26. Elliott DB. The Glenn A. Fry award lecture 2013: blurred vision, spectacle correction, and falls in older adults. Optom Vis Sci Sci. 2014;91(6):593–601.

27. Lam N, Leat SJ. Barriers to accessing low-vision care: The patient's perspective. Can J Ophthalmol. 2013;48(6).

28. Rabiee P, Parker G, Bernard S, Baxter K. Vision Rehabilitation Services: What is the evidence? University of York; 2015. p. 1–301.

29. Binns AM, Bunce C V., Dickinson CM, Harper R, Tudor-Edwards R, Woodhouse M, et al. How effective is low vision service provision? A systematic review. Surv Ophthalmol. 2012 Jan;57(1):34–65.

30. Ryan B, McCloughan L. Our better vision: what people need from low vision services in the UK. Royal National Institute of Blind People. 1999.

31. Ryan B. Models of low vision care: past, present and future. Clin Exp Optom. 2014;97(3):209–13.

Index

A

B

C

T

Printed in Great Britain
by Amazon

66906419R00132